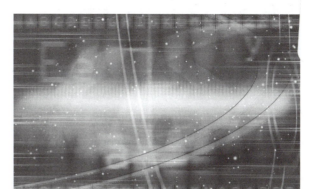

READING AND DEAFNESS: THEORY, RESEARCH, AND PRACTICE

BEVERLY J. TREZEK, Ph.D.
DePaul University

YE WANG, Ph.D.
Missouri State University

PETER V. PAUL, Ph.D.
Ohio State University

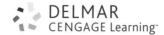
DELMAR
CENGAGE Learning™

Australia • Brazil • Japan • Korea • Mexico • Singapore • Spain • United Kingdom • United States

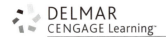

DELMAR
CENGAGE Learning

Reading and Deafness:
Theory Research and Practice
Beverly J. Trezek, Ph.D.
Ye Wang, Ph.D.
Peter V. Paul, Ph.D.

Vice President, Career and
Professional Editorial:
Dave Garza

Director of Learning Solutions:
Matthew Kane

Senior Acquisitions Editor:
Sherry Dickinson

Managing Editor:
Marah Bellegarde

Product Manager:
Laura Wood

Vice President, Career and
Professional Marketing:
Jennifer McAvey

Marketing Director: Wendy
Mapstone

Senior Marketing Manager:
Kristin McNary

Marketing Coordinator:
Scott Chrysler

Production Director:
Carolyn Miller

Production Manager:
Andrew Crouth

Content Project Manager:
Thomas Heffernan

Senior Art Director:
David Arsenault

Production Technology Analyst:
Thomas Stover

For product information and technology assistance, contact us at
Professional & Career Group Customer Support, 1-800-648-7450

For permission to use material from this text or product, submit all requests online at **www.cengage.com/permissions.**
Further permissions questions can be e-mailed to
permissionrequest@cengage.com.

Library of Congress Control Number: 2008943438

ISBN 13: 978-1-4283-2435-0

ISBN 10: 1-4283-2435-6

Delmar
5 Maxwell Drive
Clifton Park, NY 12065-2919
USA

Cengage Learning products are represented in Canada by Nelson Education, Ltd.

For your lifelong learning solutions, visit **delmar.cengage.com**

Visit our corporate website at **cengage.com**

Notice to the Reader
Publisher does not warrant or guarantee any of the products described herein or perform any independent analysis in connection with any of the product information contained herein. Publisher does not assume, and expressly disclaims, any obligation to obtain and include information other than that provided to it by the manufacturer. The reader is expressly warned to consider and adopt all safety precautions that might be indicated by the activities described herein and to avoid all potential hazards. By following the instructions contained herein, the reader willingly assumes all risks in connection with such instructions. The publisher makes no representations or warranties of any kind, including but not limited to, the warranties of fitness for particular purpose or merchantability, nor are any such representations implied with respect to the material set forth herein, and the publisher takes no responsibility with respect to such material. The publisher shall not be liable for any special, consequential, or exemplary damages resulting, in whole or part, from the readers' use of, or reliance upon, this material.

Printed in Canada
2 3 4 5 xx 10 09

CONTENTS

CHAPTER 2

COGNITIVE INTERACTIVE VIEW OF READING AND INSTRUCTION FOR STUDENTS WHO ARE DEAF OR HARD OF HEARING   26

PART 3   INSTRUCTIONAL PRACTICES

CHAPTER 4

PHONEMIC AWARENESS AND PHONICS   76

CHAPTER 5

FLUENCY 100

CHAPTER 6

VOCABULARY 120

CHAPTER 7

PART 4 IMPLICATIONS AND RECOMMENDATIONS

CHAPTER 8

READING AND LITERATE THOUGHT 166

LIST OF TABLES

PREFACE

We are proud to present this text—*Reading and Deafness: Theory, Research, and Practice*—to our readers. The context of this book reflects not only the experiences of the authors, but also our countless interactions with many talented teachers, administrators, teacher educators, and researchers working in the field of deaf education. We have divided our discussion of reading and deafness into four parts. The first part, "Theory and Research," encompasses the first three chapters. In Chapter 1, we provide an overview of reading and deafness and introduce the framework that will guide our discussion of reading for students who are deaf or hard of hearing throughout the remainder of the text. The primary goal of Chapter 2 is to introduce the reader to Chall's stages of reading development and the findings of the National Reading Panel; these serve as the theoretical and research foundations for the book. The main purpose of Chapter 3 is to explore the research on phonology and deafness. Understanding the information presented in this chapter is critically important in recognizing the application of the findings of the National Reading Panel to instructional practices for students who are deaf or hard of hearing.

The second part of the book titled "Case Studies" introduces the reader to four students who are deaf or hard of hearing. We provide the following five points of information for each student: (1) demographic information, (2) degree of hearing loss, (3) type of communication system, (4) academic history and present level of performance in reading, and (5) other relevant information. These case studies are then integrated into the third section of the book focusing on instructional practices.

"Instructional Practices" is the third part of the book and spans Chapters 4 through 7. Each chapter provides a thorough overview of the findings of the National Reading Panel in five reading curricular areas: phonemic awareness, phonics, fluency, vocabulary, and comprehension. These chapters also provide a synthesis of the research available in the field of reading and deafness to explore the alignment between the recommendations of the panel and the instructional strategies currently being utilized with students who are deaf or hard of hearing. Of particular interest to future and current teachers are the features specifically related to classroom instruction for each area such as a list of assessments, sample Individualized Education Program (IEP) goals and short-term objectives, an overview of commercially available curricula, and ideas for instructional activities.

The fourth and final part of this book, "Implications and Recommendations," includes Chapters 8 and 9. Chapter 8 introduces the readers to the concept of literate thought and explores three types of literacies: script, caption, and performance. Examples of activities that incorporate these different types of literacies into reading instruction for students who are deaf or hard of hearing are also included. In the final chapter of the book, Chapter 9, the National Reading Panel's recommendations in the areas of computer technology and teacher education are reviewed as well as relevant research in these same areas from the field of reading and deafness. The book concludes with an Epilogue that summarizes the text and offers a conclusion and directions for future research.

This book is dedicated to the current and future deaf educators who diligently seek information regarding research-based reading instructional practices and the techniques for implementing these strategies with students. We would also like to recognize the students in the Reading Specialist program at DePaul University whose creative suggestions led to many of the ideas for instructional activities offered throughout this text.

FOR THE INSTRUCTOR

An online companion is available for instructors that contains bonus materials including:

- Power Point presentations for each chapter. Use for in-class lectures and/or as lecture hand outs.

- Instructional Ideas to enhance a student's overall learning experience. Ideas include classroom and long term individual and group papers and projects, a sample grading rubric, and sample case report templates.

- Answers to the 40 Review Questions contained in the text.

Log on to http://www.delmarlearning.com/companions to access these materials.

ABOUT THE AUTHORS

Dr. Beverly J. Trezek, Ph.D. Assistant Professor, DePaul University—School of Education

Dr. Beverly Trezek received her doctorate in special education from the University of Wisconsin–Madison. Dr. Trezek has more than 12 years of experience working as a cross-categorical special education teacher and a teacher for students who are deaf or hard of hearing in the K–12 public school setting. Her research interests focus on reading instruction for beginning and struggling readers with a particular emphasis on investigating the role that phonemic awareness and phonics play in the development of reading skills for children who are deaf or hard of hearing. Dr. Trezek has recently published articles in *Journal of Deaf Studies and Deaf Education, American Annals of the Deaf, Behavioral Disorders, The Clearing House, Theory into Practice, Journal of Balanced Reading Instruction,* and *International Journal of Inclusive Education.*

Dr. Ye Wang, Ph.D. Assistant Professor, Missouri State University—Communication Sciences and Disorder

Dr. Wang received both her master's and doctoral degrees in deaf education from Ohio State University. Dr. Wang is a CODA (child of deaf adults). Her major research interest is the language and literacy development of students who are deaf or hard of hearing. Dr. Wang has recently published articles in the following prestigious journals: *Educational Researcher, Journal of Deaf Studies and Deaf Education, Theory into Practice, American Annals of the Deaf,* and *Journal of Balanced Reading Instruction.*

Dr. Peter V. Paul, Ph.D. Professor, Ohio State University—College of Education and Human Ecology

Dr. Peter V. Paul received his doctorate in interdisciplinary studies in hearing impairment from the University of Illinois, Champaign–Urbana. In addition to his position in the College of Education, Dr. Paul also holds an adjunct professorship in the Department of Speech and Hearing Science at Ohio State University. One of his major responsibilities is teacher education for individuals interested in the education of students who are deaf or hard of hearing. Dr. Paul's research interests involve the areas of vocabulary, language, and reading. He has published extensively (journals articles, chapters, books, and educational materials) on language and literacy development with respect to children who are deaf and hard of hearing. His scholarly texts include *Education and Deafness* (1990), *Toward a Psychology of Deafness* (1993), *Literacy and Deafness* (1998), and *Language and Deafness* (2001, 3rd ed.; 4th edition forthcoming). Dr. Paul has conducted workshops for educators and parents at the international, national, and state levels in the areas of literacy and literate thought. Dr. Paul has a bilateral, profound hearing impairment and is the father of a son, Peter Ben, who has Down syndrome and autism.

ACKNOWLEDGMENTS

Delmar Cengage Learning would like to extend appreciation to the following reviewers who donated their time and expertise during the development of this text:

Sandy Bowen, Ph.D.
Assistant Professor
University of Northern Colorado
Greeley, Colorado

Matthew W. D. Dye, Ph.D.
Research Associate in Brain and Cognitive Sciences
University of Rochester
Rochester, New York

Linda Jones-Oleson M.S., CCC/SLP
Speech-Language Pathologist, Supervisor
Virginia School for the Deaf and Blind
Staunton, Virginia

Lisle Kauffman, Ph.D.
Assistant Professor of Special Education
Minot State University
Minot, North Dakota

Alfred H. White, Jr., Ph.D.
Professor and Department Chair
Texas Woman's University
Denton, Texas

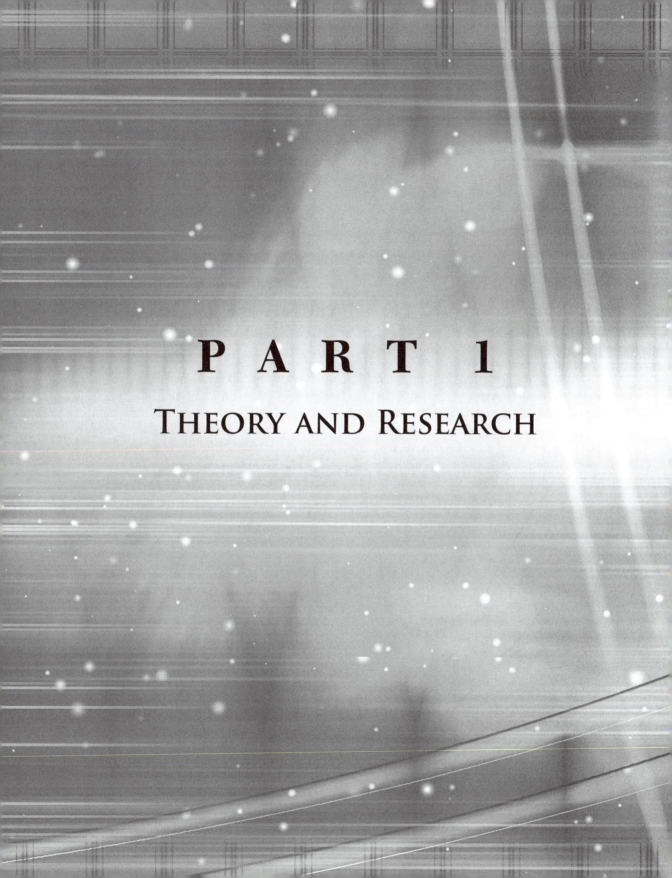

PART 1

THEORY AND RESEARCH

CHAPTER 1

INTRODUCTION TO READING AND DEAFNESS

"Is reading different for deaf individuals?" The answer appears to be both yes and no. Clearly the answer is yes in the sense that deaf readers will bring to the task of reading very different sets of language experiences than the hearing child. These differences will require special instruction. But the answer is also no. The evidence indicates that skilled deaf readers use their knowledge of the structure of English when reading. Although sign coding, in theory, might be used as an alternative to phonological coding for deaf signers, the research using various short-term memory and reading tasks has found little evidence that words are processed with references to sign by the better deaf readers. Rather, the better deaf readers, like the better hearing readers, have learned to abstract phonological information from the orthography, despite congenital and profound hearing impairment (Hanson, 1989, p. 85).

CHAPTER OBJECTIVES

After completing this chapter, the reader will be able to:

- Identify the various degrees of hearing loss
- Explain the reading achievement and comprehension levels of students who are deaf or hard of hearing
- Describe the role of reading assessment in determining levels of reading comprehension skill
- Apply the concepts of *process* and *knowledge* to explain reading difficulties
- Understand the reciprocal relationships between the conversation (spoken or signed) and written forms of English

INTRODUCTION

The passage at the beginning of this chapter exemplifies the nature and range of topics that are discussed here and in the remainder of the text. In fact, the answer to the question, Is reading different for deaf individuals? reflects perspectives on reading achievement and comprehension, descriptions of reading difficulties, relations of communication systems (e.g., **Cued Speech**, **Signing Exact English**) to reading development, the application of mainstream theories (e.g., Chall's stage theory), and recommendations for practice (e.g., findings of the National Reading Panel). What may not be obvious is that the answer also influences views on the reading development of English as a second language and the psychological reality of an entity such as **Deaf epistemology**—that is, a worldview or knowledge framework that is uniquely attributed to deaf individuals, which is analogous to the notion of a feminist epistemology (see discussion in Brueggemann, 2004, and the review by Paul, 2005).

As modest scholars, we do not propose that there is a final answer with no room for further inquiry. Rather, we argue that the dual nature (yes and no) of Hanson's answer is still tenable after almost 20 years of research and is more robust than the either–or (yes or no) answer (e.g., see Paul, 1998, 2003). As is demonstrated in this chapter, the dual nature vindicates the judicious use of mainstream theories and recommendations for literacy practice and the need to devote attention to the specific language issues of individuals who are deaf or hard of hearing. It encourages theorists and researchers to strive for a better understanding of the similarities and differences between readers who are typical and those who are not because of such conditions as deafness or other disabilities.

Those who espouse a predominately yes answer to Hanson's question seem to argue for a Deaf epistemology or, rather, seem to assert that the reading acquisition process of deaf individuals is so radically different that we cannot and should not use mainstream theories and practices. The assumption is that deaf individuals are visual learners or must use their vision to learn. Thus, for example, the development and implementation of practices (e.g., phonemic awareness activities and use of phonics) based on the research of hearing children who hear and speak are meaningless and inappropriate (see reviews in Musselman, 2000; Paul, 2003). There is also the assumption that deaf children and adolescents think differently from hearing individuals and, thus, these individuals use nonphonological means (e.g., signs, finger spelling) for comprehending a printed text. In essence, with respect to the research on phonological coding (see Chapter 3 of this text), the assumption is that deaf readers can bypass this component by using orthography or other means or by going straight from print to meaning.

How does this work? To put it simplistically for now, let us consider the following short passage:

A woman needs a man like a fish needs a bicycle. In this postmodern age, it is becoming clear that a number of women do not feel the need to be married or attached to be whole or even to have children.

It is not necessary to have a man or even a father in the household.

[*Note:* First sentence is taken from Gough, 1984, p. 225].

Proponents might argue that deaf children convert print to signs (preferably from **American Sign Language (ASL)***) or* **finger spelling** *to decode this passage and to arrive at the meaning. That is, the act of decoding means a representation of the words (or letters) via the use of signs or finger spelling. After this conversion, meaning is negotiated or constructed in the head. In this view, deaf individuals cannot or do not use a phonological code (pronunciation or inner speech) to convert letters to sounds and then work out the meaning in the head.*

Within this view, it is sometimes presumed that students do not need an explicit understanding of the structure of English or do not need explicit lessons in English in order to learn to read English. Meaning can be explained or negotiated via the use of American Sign Language only in conjunction with English print. This is the predominate basis for using ASL to teach English as a second language. Specifically, it is the use of ASL to explain the words or sentences in English print. In this view, there is no manipulation of the primary form (speech or signs) of English or even the need to learn such entities (see discussions in Paul, 1998, 2001).

Proponents of a predominately no answer to Hanson's question argue that English reading is basically the same for everyone. It does not matter whether you have a learning disability or are learning English as a second language, there are certain fundamentals that are critical for the acquisition of reading in English including an understanding of the structure (grammar) of English. From one perspective, these fundamentals are similar (or may be similar in the strong sense) to what has been proposed by the National Reading Panel (NRP) (2000)—that is, phonemic awareness, phonics, fluency, vocabulary, and comprehension instruction. The no answer also implies that deaf or hard of hearing readers, whether reading English as a first or second language, make errors, use strategies, and proceed through stages that are roughly developmentally similar to native English users reading English as a first language (e.g., see reviews in Hanson, 1989; Paul, 1998). And, as indicated by Hanson (1989) in the quote at the beginning of this chapter, the better deaf readers seem to use a phonological code and are knowledgeable about the structure of English.

Consequently, it can be argued that the acquisition of reading by children and adolescents who are deaf or hard of hearing is qualitatively similar to that of native first-language readers of English. Because of this, it has been recently averred that there is or may be merit in applying the recommendations of the National Reading Panel to readers who are deaf or hard of hearing (Schirmer & McGough, 2005). In addition, there is a growing body of research showing not only that the use of a phonological code via a development of phonemic awareness and phonic skills is important for beginning reading skill, but also that it is possible for deaf or hard of hearing students to learn about phonological and phonemic awareness, especially via the use of **Visual Phonics** *(Trezek & Malmgren, 2005; Trezek & Wang, 2006; Trezek, Wang, Woods, Gampp, & Paul, 2007; see also Chapters 3 and 4 of this text).*

Admittedly, we believe that a synthesis of the research on children reading English as a first or second language has strongly supported a predominantly no answer to Hanson's question (e.g., see reviews in Paul, 1998, 2001, 2003), but we are sensitive to the implications of the yes part of the answer. For example, we recognize that many adolescents who are deaf or hard of hearing would have difficulties understanding the passage presented previously because of additional challenges associated with language and experience (e.g., prior knowledge, metacognition). Even if students can decode the passage nicely, they would have enormous comprehension problems with, for example, the figurative usage and comparison in the first sentence (A woman needs a man like a fish needs a bicycle), the syntax (word order) in the second and third sentences (e.g., the use of phrases such as, it is becoming or it is not necessary), and selected vocabulary of both function (e.g., in this; in the) and content words (e.g., postmodern age and household).

These constructions in the examples above may also cause problems for readers who are hearing. Nevertheless, on the whole, students who are deaf or hard of hearing have more difficulties with the components of language (morphology, syntax, etc.) than do hearing counterparts. The yes part of the answer to Hanson's question indicates that, for many children and adolescents who are deaf or hard of hearing, learning to read is both a language (in the broad sense) and a reading issue. It is critical, at least, to improve the understanding of the structure of English by children who are deaf or hard of hearing so this can aid in the development of reading skills. So, for us, we argue that there is a predominately no answer to Hanson's question, but we need to be sensitive to the yes aspects, particularly as they relate to language and experience.

The plan for this chapter is as follows. First, we provide a description of deafness so that our readers can be informed of the characteristics of individuals for whom the information in this text is applicable. We will then discuss a general overview of the reading achievement of students who are deaf or hard of hearing and present a few salient reasons for this current level. We investigate how reading achievement of students who are deaf or hard of hearing has been measured and present a process-and-knowledge view as the framework for understanding the reading difficulties of these children and adolescents. We summarize the chapter by introducing the rationale for the present text.

DESCRIPTION OF DEAFNESS

It should be clear that there is no one definition or description of deafness. Deafness has been defined in a variety of ways, often influenced by the educational and professional experiences of individuals who attempt to provide descriptions. We will follow a simple approach here—that is, our description is mostly audiometric.

Hearing impairment is a generic term referring to all types, causes, and degree of hearing loss. An individual's hearing threshold level is indicated on the audiogram as a *pure-tone average* (PTA), unaided, across a range of speech frequencies (500, 1000, 2000 Hertz). The pure-tone audiogram is designed to chart hearing sensitivity from 0 dB to 110 dB (see discussions in Ross, 1986; Schow & Nerbonne,

2007). The categories of hearing impairment and educational implications are illustrated in Table 1-1.

With respect to Table 1-1, the reader should keep in mind that these are general educational implications associated with degrees of hearing impairment. There are, of course, individual variations that may be affected, for example, age at onset of hearing loss (i.e., before or after 2 years of age) or other factors such as familial influences, IQ, and socioeconomic status. Individuals with hearing impairment up to, but not including, the severe category level are often labeled **hard of hearing,** whereas those in the severe to profound categories are often labeled **deaf**. These labels refer to audiometric characteristics (i.e., with respect to hearing status). It is possible for an individual in the severe impairment category, for example,

to *function* like a hard of hearing person in the areas of language and literacy even though she or he may be audiometrically deaf (Paul, 2001; Schow & Nerbonne, 2007).

This text is mostly concerned with individuals in the severe to profound categories (i.e., 70 dB to 89 dB and 90 dB +); however, many of the concepts and instructional strategies included in our discussions are also applicable to students who are considered hard of hearing. Nevertheless, students with severe to profound hearing losses are those who most likely will need alternative methods, such as Cued Speech and Visual Phonics, to develop aspects of reading such as phonological and phonemic awareness. In addition, it is also critical to expend a substantial amount of time on higher-level reading skills such as vocabulary, prior knowledge, and metacognition. All

TABLE 1-1 Categories of Hearing Loss and Educational Implications

Degree of Hearing Loss	Description	Implications
Up to 26 decibels	Normal	No special classes or treatment.
27 to 40 decibels	Slight	Does not typically require special class or treatment. May need instruction in lip reading and speech. May need amplification. May need assistance in language or reading.
41 to 54 decibels	Mild	May need special class or school placement. Requires instruction in lip reading and speech. Requires instruction in the use of hearing aids. Requires special assistance in language or reading.
55 to 69 decibels	Moderate	May require special class or school placement. Requires instruction in lip reading and speech. Requires instruction in the use of hearing aids. Requires special instruction in language or reading.
70 to 89 decibels	Severe	Requires a full-time special education program with special instruction in language and reading. Needs comprehensive support services and training in lip reading, speech, and the use of residual hearing.
90 decibels or greater	Profound	Requires a full-time special education program with special instruction in language and reading. Needs comprehensive support services and training in lip reading, speech, and the use of residual hearing. Usually requires the use of sign communication.

Note: Some scholars (e.g., Schow & Nerboone, 2007) have argued that there should be two sets of categories for slight and mild—one for children and one for adults—although there is little difference between these two sets. Others argue that the slight impairment category should begin at 15 or 16 dB, instead of 27 dB (e.g., Ross, 1986).
Source: Adapted from Moores (2001), Ross (1986), and Schow & Nerbonne (2007).

of these reading variables are discussed later in this chapter.

READING ACHIEVEMENT AND DEAFNESS

Much of what we know about reading achievement is based on standardized reading achievement surveys, particularly those that assess general achievement with subtests pertaining to literacy. In general, it is well documented that most students with severe to profound hearing impairment do not read as well as their hearing counterparts upon graduation from high school (see reviews in Allen, 1986; Moores, 2006; Paul, 2003; Schirmer & McGough, 2005; Traxler, 2000). Even more interesting, these results have not changed much since the beginning of the use of standardized tests to measure reading achievement levels (see discussions in Marschark, 2007; Rose, McAnally, & Quigley, 2004; Quigley & Paul, 1986). Two persistent, general patterns have been frequently documented: (1) average 18- to 19-year-old students with severe to profound hearing impairment are reading no better than average 9- to 10-year-old hearing students, and (2) there seems to be an annual growth rate of less than a half grade per year with a leveling off or plateau effect occurring at the third- or fourth-grade level for most students.

What are the reasons for the above, persistent findings, which often cause quite a bit of anguish for both parents and teachers? Similar to any other complex entity, and considering the difficulties of conducting research on a low-incidence population such as deafness, the reasons are neither simple nor straightforward. Only a few remarks are made here.

Paul (2001) proffered the following factors as a partial explanation of these general findings (see also McGuinness, 2004, 2005; Pearson, 2004, for a discussion of factors for children who are hearing):

- It is possible that the low reading scores are the results of artifacts associated with the type of test used to measure reading achievement. That is, different aspects of tests (e.g., use of multiple-choice questions, cloze procedures, language of distracters) might produce different results. Ironically, this condition could lead to an overestimation of the actual reading levels of the students (e.g., Davey, LaSasso, & Macready, 1983; Moores, 2001).

- The inferential (e.g., answering questions, drawing conclusion) and language (e.g., difficulty of syntax, figurative language) demands of reading materials increase dramatically after the third-grade level. These demands exhibit their greatest deleterious effects on students who are at risk at the end of second or third grade. That is, students who are behind by the end of second or third grade find it difficult to deal with the increased cognitive and linguistic demands of advanced reading texts (see also the discussions in McGuinness, 2004; Pearson, 2004; Snowling & Hulme, 2005).

- Many students with severe to profound hearing impairment have marked difficulty in developing or acquiring the language of print (i.e., English). In other words, these students do not possess a working, intuitive knowledge of the components of English such as phonology (e.g., consonants, vowels), morphology (e.g., word parts such as -ing, -ment, or in-), syntax (word order), and semantics (meanings of words and phrases). In essence, students have both processing (i.e., identification of letters or words) and knowledge (e.g., prior, background, or world knowledge; metacognition) problems. This results in a breakdown of the reciprocity between the conversational (spoken or signed) and written forms of the language of print (see also the discussions in McGuinness, 2004, 2005; Paul, 2003; Snowling & Hulme, 2005).

- Teachers of students who are deaf or hard of hearing may not be adequately prepared by their university-level teacher-education programs to teach reading (or writing) in the schools. That is, teachers may not have had a sufficient amount of reading education courses or have not been shown how to adapt (e.g., differentiate instruction) what they have learned to meet the needs of children and adolescents who are deaf or hard of hearing. With respect to the areas of the National Reading Panel (2000) discussed later in this text, it is possible that teachers have not received enough education in the importance and application of such National Reading Panel aspects as phonemic awareness, phonics, vocabulary, fluency, and comprehension.

Given the difficulty of reading for many students who are deaf or hard of hearing, it is not uncommon for teachers to develop an impassioned, biased allegiance to a specific philosophy (e.g., whole language), use of specific materials (e.g., children's literature), or even a specific instructional strategy (e.g., phonics, whole word). In addition, teachers and parents might presume that there is a strong, unitary, one-dimensional relationship between reading achievement and the type of communication form used during early childhood or during the early childhood period. Specifically, there is the belief that a specific communication system such as **oralism**, Signing Exact English, **Seeing Essential English**, or American Sign Language that leads directly to the development of beginning and advanced reading skills in English (e.g.,

see discussion in Paul, 2001). As discussed in the ensuing chapters of this text, many of the above assertions regarding the communication systems and other instructional issues are not supported by research. In addition, there may be a strong need to improve the quality and type of reading instructional strategies that preservice teachers learn in teacher education or deaf education programs in university settings.

UNDERSTANDING READING ASSESSMENT AND READING ACHIEVEMENT

To shed more light on these issues, a couple of fundamental questions need to be addressed: (1) How has reading achievement been measured? and (2) What do we mean by achievement? With respect to the first question, we are interested in the types of assessments that have been used to evaluate reading ability in children and adolescents who are deaf or hard of hearing. On one hand, the answer to the second question is related to that of the first question. However, this is not as simple as it looks, especially if we intend achievement to be synonymous with comprehension (see discussion in Pearson & Hamm, 2005).

Assessment and Reading

How has reading achievement been measured? Similar to the situation in the larger field of reading and hearing children (Pearson & Hamm, 2005), the manner in which reading has been assessed in children who are deaf or hard of hearing has been influenced by the prevailing thinking of the times (Paul, 1998; Paul & Jackson, 1993). Of course, an additional influence can be seen in what can be called the *language-dominant hypothesis* (from the field of linguistic) in which a predominant amount of focus for explaining reading (and other entities) was placed on the use and development of language. Indeed, most teachers of children who are deaf or hard of hearing think of themselves as *language teachers,* and many of the reading difficulties of children who are deaf or hard of hearing have been attributed to their overall English language comprehension problems. That is, the reading achievement levels were a reflection of the inadequate development of the English language.

This heavy reliance on language can be seen in the types of tests used during the early part of the 20th century to measure reading achievement. The exemplar is the use of the cloze procedure in which every *n*th (3rd, 4th, 5th, etc.) word is omitted (e.g., Pintner, 1918, 1927). Examples of test items are as follows:

We like good boys _____ girls.

The _____ is barking at the car.

This reliance on language was also evident in items that focus on students' understanding of the language of the test. Examples follow:

How many ears has a cat?

Put a question mark after this sentence.

Another common way to assess reading ability was the use of standardized achievement tests such as the Metropolitan and Stanford tests. The reading score was the combined score associated with two subtests: *Word Meaning* and *Paragraph Meaning* (e.g., Balow, Fulton, & Peploe, 1971; Wrightstone, Aronow, & Moskowitz, 1963). The Word Meaning subtest is essentially a vocabulary test whereas the Paragraph Meaning subtest involves the use of a brief passage with questions and alternatives presented in a multiple-choice format. The use of sentences or short passages or the reliance on vocabulary subsets (i.e., word meaning) as an evaluation of reading ability continued throughout the 1970s and 1980s for

both students who were hearing and deaf or hard of hearing (Paul, 1998; Pearson & Hamm, 2005).

Prior to the 1970s, nearly all of the formal standardized or achievement tests used with students who were deaf or hard of hearing were normed on hearing students. That is, in developing these tests, students who were deaf or hard of hearing were not part of the normative or test sample. This resulted in charges that these tests were not valid or were inappropriate, especially with respect to some of the items, because they involved the use of hearing. A good example is the labeling or recognition of similar or dissimilar sounds in words (e.g., see discussion in Babbini & Quigley, 1970).

From the late 1960s to the 1980s, an adapted version of the Stanford Achievement Test (SAT) was developed, administered to, and normed on samples of students who were deaf or hard of hearing (Allen, 1986; Qi & Mitchell, 2007; Traxler, 2000; Trybus & Karchmer, 1977). It was then possible to compare the scores of students who were deaf or hard of hearing to those of hearing counterparts in a more valid and reliable manner. In addition, during the 1980s, criterion-referenced tests began to emerge and markedly influenced the assessment of reading (Pearson & Hamm, 2005). Criterion-referenced tests are used to diagnose the strengths and weaknesses of the individuals in specific critical areas (e.g., vocabulary, answering inferential questions). This movement produced tests that can be used not only to diagnose reading difficulties, but also to make judgments of overall achievement (i.e., standardized) levels.

Some common reading standardized tools or *formal* tests used with hearing students with potential for use with students who are deaf or hard of hearing can be found in several sources (e.g., Bradley-Johnson & Evans, 1991; Farr & Carey, 1986; King & Quigley, 1985; Lipson & Wixson, 1997; McCormick, 1987; Schirmer, 1994). The above sources also contain a good discussion of the advantages and disadvantages of using these tests.

Informal assessments were also used, and these refer to the use of tests such as the cloze procedures (discussed previously), informal reading inventories (e.g., Informal Reading Inventory [IRI]), Reading Miscue Inventory (RMI), and placement and end-of-level tests associated with reading series (see King & Quigley, 1985, for a discussion of advantages and disadvantages). Informal reading inventories might be a useful tool for providing some information on the strengths and weaknesses of students who are deaf or hard of hearing—for example, word identification, vocabulary, and comprehension. That is, they can provide some information similar to the more formal diagnostic or criterion-referenced tests (for a detailed discussion of common IRIs and diagnostic assessments, see Farr & Carey, 1986; McCormick, 1987).

As indicated previously, regardless of the type of test used—formal or informal—the overall reading achievement level of most students who are deaf and a number of hard of hearing seem to plateau or level off at the third- or fourth-grade level (Paul, 2003; Qi & Mitchell, 2007; Traxler, 2000). In one sense, a slow growth rate is reflective of this plateau. However, the growth rate is uneven: There does not always seem to be a steady progress from year to year for many children and adolescents who are deaf or hard of hearing. It is typical to find that some children are at a certain reading level in one year and then seem to lose ground (i.e., enter a lower reading level) the next year. This might result from the difficulty of measuring reading achievement, artifacts of the tests, or other factors that have not been delineated (e.g., see discussions in Ewoldt, 1987; Moores, 1996).

To make matters more distressing—so to speak—it has been argued that the general achievement batteries might be overestimating the reading achievement levels (Davey et al.,

1983; Moores, 1996). This means that the actual levels might be lower than those reported. Nevertheless, these general findings have been documented since the beginning of the formal testing movement in the early 1900s (deVilliers, 1991; Quigley & Paul, 1986). To reiterate an earlier point, there is no question that language is important for reading. Specifically, it is the reciprocal relation between the conversational (spoken or signed) form of the language and the language of print that is crucial (Adams, 1990, 1994; McGuinness, 2004, 2005; Snow, Burns, & Griffin, 1998; Templeton & Bear, 1992). This reciprocal relation presents challenges with respect to the use of sign systems of English, a system such as Cued Speech, or even the use of ASL in a bilingual–bicultural situation as is discussed briefly later in this chapter.

Meanwhile, there is more to reading than language development. We also argue and show in this text that, for many students who are deaf or hard of hearing, particularly poor readers, it is necessary to teach reading skills explicitly in meaningful, structured situations (e.g., Adams, 1990, 1994; National Reading Panel, 2000; Pearson, 2004; Snow et al., 1998). In order for this to be effective or successful, teachers need to be well informed about the nature and instruction of reading. This deep knowledge of reading enables the teacher to be creative in selecting alternative strategies to replace ineffective ones in the teaching of reading. We return to this issue in the ensuing chapters of this text.

Comprehension and Reading

Many reading scholars would answer our second question—What is reading achievement?—by responding that it is a measure of reading comprehension (e.g., Paris & Stahl, 2005). That is, the predominant focus should be on comprehension, which drives the development of adequate assessment materials. Within this view, there is no denial of the importance of variables such as phonemic awareness or vocabulary, which are important areas for instruction. The bulk of the attention, however, should be on comprehension for understanding reading achievement. Other scholars, promoting what is often called a **Simple View of Reading** (e.g., Gough & Tunmer, 1986), argue for assessing word recognition, phonemic awareness, and text comprehension of narrative and expository passages (e.g., Catts & Kamhi, 2005). Much of the focus of the Simple View is on decoding and text comprehension—areas that should be assessed and should be the main foci of instruction. The Simple View seems to emphasize the accessing and comprehension of a single passage (i.e., passage-specific information), whereas a broader view is concerned with factors such as prior knowledge (topic *and* broad knowledge), metacognition, and attitude (engagement), which can impact both decoding and comprehension. The broader view advocates the use of several passages on comprehension tests.

Reading comprehension has been measured in several ways and has also been influenced by the prevailing thinking of the times (Pearson & Hamm, 2005). There has been a paradigmatic shift in the views on reading comprehension, and this shift—called a *revolutionary shift*—seems to have emerged during the late 1970s with the advent of cognitive theories of reading.

To understand this change, it might be best to discuss a few of the shortcomings of the types of reading comprehension tests that have been used and, for the most part, remain in use today (Pearson & Hamm, 2005; Pearson & Stallman, 1994; Pearson & Valencia, 1986). In addition, we need to highlight a few assessment issues related to children and adolescents who are deaf or hard of hearing. Finally, we end with a discussion of the concept of *comprehension,* a term that can be operationally defined but, in our view, is more complex

than educators have imagined. Our goal here is to demonstrate that there is a great need to research comprehension and to develop more valid reading comprehension tests even though the concept of comprehension seems to be somewhat elusive for those who favor a broad view of reading.

Nature of Current Reading Comprehension Assessments

Several problems associated with current reading assessments have been documented in several reviews (Pearson & Hamm, 2005; Pearson & Stallman, 1994; Pearson & Valencia, 1986). Many of these problems are related to the use of one passage (often a short one) for assessment purposes. For example, even though it has been argued that prior knowledge is an important variable in reading comprehension, several of the current assessments continue to use short passages or numerous short topics that preclude or mask any relationship between prior knowledge and reading comprehension. Another criticism is the type of questions asked—most of which are fairly literal and do not require more complex inferential skills. Examples of low-level, literal questions include those focusing on sequence (e.g., what happened first, second, or third) or on specific details of the text (e.g., factual information or descriptive details such as size and color). There is a place for a few low-level literal questions, but the bulk of the questions should require readers to make inferences, apply the information to other passages, and make evaluative comments.

Asking good questions about the reading selection, as well as answering them, is a good index of expert reading skill. Nevertheless, students are rarely required to create or select questions about the selection after reading it on assessments. The predominant use of certain formats, such as multiple-choice with a single answer, do not assist students in recognizing that there could be alternative correct answers based on several or a wide variety of perspectives. Finally, this heavy focus on single passages undermines one of the most important hallmarks of a good, critical reader—one who is able to synthesize and evaluate issues after reading several passages on the same topic.

Comprehension Assessment and Deafness

With respect to students who are deaf or hard of hearing, comprehension might also be affected by the format (mentioned above) of the test, that is, the use of multiple-choice, yes–no, or even cloze procedures (e.g., for a detailed discussion of these problems, see King & Quigley, 1985; LaSasso, 1999; Moores, 1996; Paul & Quigley, 1990). A cloze procedure (omitting every *n*th word), which has been used in the early achievement tests discussed previously, is particularly problematic. One reason is that this format requires knowledge of the English language, particularly syntax and grammar, in order to complete the sentences. This specific knowledge might prevent investigators

from obtaining an accurate measure of reading comprehension because of the confounding language factor.

One of the most important caveats of using a particular format is the need to devote attention to the application of specific strategies by students who are deaf or hard of hearing during reading tasks. For example, it has been observed that students use association strategies or visual matching strategies that are prompted by the wording of the items on the tests (e.g., see discussions in LaSasso, 1985, 1999; Wolk & Schildroth, 1984). Examples of visual matching strategies are illustrated in Table 1-2.

Awareness of these and other test-taking strategies might lead to the development of test items that are more appropriate for students who are deaf or hard of hearing. More specifically, students can be shown that their incorrect answers result from the use of inappropriate or inefficient strategies (e.g., see discussion in LaSasso, 1999).

It is important also to remember the assumptions of using paper-and-pencil measures for an understanding of the reading comprehension ability of students who are deaf

TABLE 1-2 Examples of Visual Matching Strategies

Type of Strategy	Text (Sample)	Question	Answer
Response (a) does not contain key words, (b) is within the sentence that contains key words, and (c) is vertically aligned with key words.	Nature has a similar method for cooling off the body. When little particles of water, called perspiration, are evaporated from the skin, the body is cooled to 98.6 degrees.	What is perspiration composed of?	98.6 degrees
Response (a) does not contain key words, (b) is within the sentence that contains key words, (c) is neither vertically or horizontally aligned with key words, and (d) is within two lines above or below line containing key words.	The electric eel is a fish that is native to South America. It defends itself from attacks of enemies by a natural electric battery. A discharge from this battery is powerful.	How is the eel used by the Indians?	attacks of enemies

Source: Adapted from LaSasso (1985). See also the discussions in King & Quigley (1985) and LaSasso (1999).

or hard of hearing. These types of measures focus on the students' ability to understand information presented in a print mode. Specifically, reading comprehension tests require students to read and write their responses. These types of tests demand, at least, proficiency in the language in which the students are supposed to read and write. This type of mode is feasible for attempting to understand the students' ability to access and comprehend print materials—in general.

We caution the predominant use of this mode for all aspects of achievement or comprehension. As discussed in Chapter 8 of this text, it is possible that students have prior knowledge or understanding about a topic that they are unable to retrieve because of their struggles with the English language on paper-and-pencil tests. In other words, some students may know the answers to questions that are presented to them through speech or signs, but this knowledge is evident only if they are permitted to answer the questions in the same expressive, conversational mode (i.e., speech or signs). Students might not be able to demonstrate their knowledge about science or social studies or other academic areas as required by standardized tests and other similar assessments in print. Despite these assertions (see also Chapter 8), some educators maintain that "it can be argued that achievement tests measure the ability of students to understand information presented at a certain literate level in the majority language of mainstream society" (Paul & Quigley, 1990, p. 16).

The Slippery Slope of Comprehension

Regardless of what type of assessment has been used and despite the flaws of current comprehension tests, there is no doubt that many students who are deaf or hard of hearing have difficulty in demonstrating their comprehension of print materials. In addition to improving reading education programs in university *deaf education* programs, there is also a need to develop better reading comprehension tests. The issue of a better test begs the question: What is reading comprehension?

This fundamental question spawns numerous others. The list below is not exhaustive, but it captures the gist of the discussions on the proposed new directions in reading comprehension tests (e.g., Paris & Stahl, 2005).

- Is reading comprehension simply the ability to answer questions or the ability to retell the passage in your own words?

- Is it possible to answer questions and not truly understand the passage or be able to apply your understanding to other areas?

- Is retelling a good measure of reading comprehension? What are the guidelines for retelling?

- Is reading comprehension restricted to presenting one interpretation of the text or should readers address multiple interpretations and multiple perspectives?

- Should readers respond to the text—that is, develop a critical stance?

- Is comprehension affected by sociocultural or sociohistorical issues such as an author's voice or stance or the context of the times in which the story or passage was written?

Then there are issues related to genre and critical reading.

- Should reading comprehension be restricted to one type of genre—fiction, nonfiction, expository, narrative, and so on?

- Do we want children and adolescents to handle a variety of passages in formats ranging from newspapers to texts to magazines?

- Should we expect students to read critically by comparing one perspective on a controversial topic to another perspective?

It is possible that we need to move away from what can be called a Simple View of Comprehension with a predominant focus on one selection or passage to the use of several passages that includes not only the ability to demonstrate comprehension of what is read, but also the ability to proffer several layers of meanings or interpretations. It is clear that there is no single unitary comprehension process to be measured (see discussions in Paris & Stahl, 2005). Perhaps, we should ask and address this question: Comprehension of what, for what, and for whom? On one hand, we think we know quite a bit about the reading comprehension ability of children and adolescents who are deaf or hard of hearing, particularly with the use of single passages. On the other hand, what we know may be extremely limited according to the broad view of reading with the focus on what it means to be a critical reader. Nevertheless, reading comprehension is difficult with either a single passage or with multiple passages. In the next section, we present one model for viewing these difficulties with respect to children and adolescents who are deaf or hard of hearing.

PROCESS AND KNOWLEDGE

Is there a best approach for describing the reading situation of children who are deaf or hard of hearing? Can any approach address the use of the various language or communication systems? Paul (2001) proffered a framework for understanding the reading difficulties of children and adolescents who are deaf or hard of hearing that has been refined as the **process-and-knowledge view** (e.g., Paul, 2003). The process-and-knowledge view

asserts that there is a reciprocal relation between the processing of print and an understanding or interpretation of the information. The emphasis is on this reciprocity: The process domain facilitates the use of the knowledge domain, and the knowledge domain facilitates the better use of the process domain.

Processing print refers to access skills such as the use of word identification and larger discourse processes as well as the ability to convert print—typically via the use of a phonological code—for the purpose of constructing meaning in the head. There is also the processing of larger units such as phrases and sentences, which compels the reader to hold in memory (particularly in short-term or working memory; see Chapter 3) what was processed earlier in the phrase or sentence. The goal is for processing to become automatic so that much of the reader's energy and resources can be used to comprehend and interpret the text.

The knowledge domain is a broad entity. If we relate this to the Simple View of Reading (Gough & Tunmer, 1986), then this domain refers to the specific knowledge or information or skills (inferences, etc.) for answering questions about or understanding the specifics of a particular story or passage. Paul (2003) intended for this domain not only to encompass what is needed to comprehend the story or passage, but also to relate to other broad knowledge that influences the comprehension of the story as well as the extension of that comprehension to other stories. In short, the knowledge domain refers to prior knowledge of the story (including the language of print) and other broad related topics, metacognitive skills (including inferential skills), and awareness of the social and contextual frameworks of the story. The knowledge domain also includes those aspects of critical reading that were discussed previously in the section on reading comprehension—for example, taking a stance, evaluating points of views, asking questions about the story, and so on.

Let us consider the following passage.

The Reconstruction of the South after the Civil War was a mixed blessing. Depending on where you live, you were most likely to view this process as either positive or negative—beneficial or destructive. According to some scholars, this is what we should expect at the conclusion of any war. The rebuilding of the infrastructure on the losing side is fraught with controversies and, sometimes, corruption.

Now let us apply the process-and-knowledge framework to indicate how this works for the above passage. In decoding this passage, readers apply their understanding of letters and sounds (i.e., decoding processes) as well as words and sentences. This understanding is part of both the processing domain and the knowledge domain in that readers have internalized the structure of English—that is, phonology, morphology, syntax, and semantics. The visual processing (process domain) of letters provides the spark of identification and other associated processes—which are phonological, orthographic (arrangement of letters, etc.), and meaning (semantic) information. The phonological coding process is activated and assists with the relations between phonemes (sounds) and graphemes (letters). The use of phonological coding is important to hold information in memory (see Chapter 3). By the time the reader arrives at *mixed blessing,* she or he needs to remember the earlier part of that sentence—*The Reconstruction of the South. . . .* A general knowledge (knowledge domain) of the Civil War assists with the understanding of this passage; however, a general knowledge of the aftermaths of wars provides even more of a perspective, especially within a social context. In addition, readers are aware that history—or something

similar—is often presented from the framework or mind-set of a writer who also has social and contextual influences (e.g., location of residence; time period in which the history is written; etc.). Thus, readers should be able to compare a perspective of one writer with those of others on the concept of reconstruction after one war or several wars (knowledge domain).

In essence, the development of conventional reading requires processing the form (i.e., written code as in the structure of letters, words, and sentences) to construct or obtain meaning (i.e., comprehension and interpretation) and to apply it to other situations. To achieve reading fluency, readers need to reach the threshold at which word identification becomes automatic and almost effortless so that most of the energy can be spent on comprehending and interpreting the message. All readers need extensive experiences with print, which results in growths in language variables such as vocabulary, morphology, and syntax, and other variables such as knowledge of topics and culture. This growth in the knowledge domain supports the process domain and strengthens the reciprocal relations between these two domains.

Reciprocity and Second-Language Learning

It is becoming clear that the reciprocal link between the conversational and written forms of English is also critical for students learning English as a second language (e.g., see reviews in Paul, 2001 [Chapter 9]; Paul, 2003). This is, indeed, a surprising—perhaps unacceptable—finding, even for most proponents of ASL and English bilingual programs. Although it is possible for second-language learners to learn about the English culture for the purpose of reading and writing through the use of their native language, there is no compelling evidence that these students can achieve a high level of English literacy along this route. We admit that more research is needed, but this is our synthesis of the current research state. In essence, exposure to the print of a phonetic language with explanations in another language (spoken or signed) is simply not sufficient or efficient. This process precludes a reciprocal relationship that can and should exist between the conversational and written forms of the same language to be learned. Thus, in most cases, individuals need to learn to manipulate the conversational form of the language of print, especially a phonemic language such as English, in order to facilitate the understanding of information from the written form (e.g., print).

An interesting line of support for Hanson's (1989) assertion at the beginning of the chapter can be gleaned from a study conducted more than 25 years ago (King, 1981) with findings that have not been challenged substantially since that time (e.g., see discussions in Paul, 2001, 2003). King (1981) was interested in whether the acquisition of English by students who are deaf (90 decibels or greater in the better ear) was different from or similar to hearing students learning English as a first language. She was able to study students who are deaf for whom English was a first or second language and to compare her findings with students who are deaf for whom English was a first language in earlier investigations (e.g., see discussion in Russell, Quigley, & Power, 1976). King reported that both groups of students who are deaf experienced order difficulties in syntax (word order) similar to hearing students learning English as a first language. What was even more remarkable is that both groups of students who are deaf produced errors that were roughly similar. Examples of these errors made by the deaf students are illustrated in Table 1-3.

TABLE 1-3 Examples of Errors by Deaf and Hearing Students

Distinctive Structure	Environment	Example
Negative outside sentence	Negation	No Daddy see baby
Inversion of subject and object	Questions	Who TV watched?
Omission of *be* or *have*	Verbs	John sick. The girl a ball.
Confusion of tense markers	Verbs	Tom has pushing the wagon.
Third-person marker missing	Verbs	The boy say "hi."
Omission of conjunction	Conjunction	Bob saw liked the bike.
Omission of determiner	Determiner	Boy is sick.
Confusion of determiners	Determiner	The some apples.
Confusion of case pronouns	Pronouns	Her is going home.

Note: Adapted from King (1981).

Thus, King (1981) and others (e.g., Hayes & Arnold, 1992; Paul, 1998, 2001, 2003) offered the following findings:

- In general, the acquisition of English as a second language by students who are deaf or hard of hearing is developmentally similar to the acquisition of English by native users who are hearing.

- The acquisition of English as a first language by children and adolescents who are deaf or hard of hearing is developmentally similar to the acquisition of English by native users who are hearing.

- Whether learning English as a first or second language, students who are deaf or hard of hearing produce errors, use strategies, or proceed through stages that are roughly similar to younger hearing individuals learning English as a first language. Of course, there are individual differences and a few esoteric patterns; however, the bulk of evidence seems to support a qualitative-similarity hypothesis (i.e., similar developmental patterns).

- The reciprocity between the conversational (spoken or signed) and written (print) forms of English is operable for learning English as a first or second language.

In our view, the findings above, particularly the reciprocity principle, indirectly substantiates the use of the recommendations of the National Reading Panel (2000) for children and adolescents who are deaf or hard of hearing. A similar argument has also been made by others (e.g., Schirmer & McGough, 2005).

Reciprocity and the Use of Communication Systems

A persistent, controversial issue in the field of deafness has been the effects of the English sign systems and other communication systems (e.g., Cued Speech/Language) on the development of English reading skills (e.g., see reviews in Moores, 1996; Paul, 2001). Does the reciprocity principle apply to students who are deaf or hard of hearing exposed to any of the above communication systems? Not only is the answer *yes*, but also it can be related to the importance of phonemic awareness—indeed phonology and morphology—for beginning reading skills.

With respect to the various communication systems such as signed English (Bornstein, Saulnier, & Hamiliton, 1983), Signing Exact English (Gustason & Zawolkow, 1993), Seeing Essential English (Anthony, 1966), and Cued Speech/Language (Fleetwood & Metzger, 1998), a few students who are deaf or hard of

hearing do acquire a level of competency in English, but the reasons for this phenomenon are not completely clear. It has been suggested that one major reason is the degree of access to English phonology, which is considered to be one of the building blocks of a language—any language (e.g., Fleetwood & Metzger, 1998; Paul, 2001, 2003). This access seems to be the result of students' attempts to understand and produce speech (e.g., simultaneous communication, speech reading, Cued Speech) and of their abstractions of phonologic and orthographic information from reading and writing English. Eventually, along with other important variables in reading, this leads to an understanding of the alphabetic principle, the system on which English reading is based. The acquisition and development of phonology and phonemic awareness are issues discussed further in Chapters 3 and 4 of this text.

Regardless of the theoretical underpinnings, there seems to be sufficient evidence that students who are deaf or hard of hearing, as well as other students, need to understand the connection between the phonemes of a phonetic language and the graphemes of print, especially for a language such as English. There needs to be an awareness that English speech can be segmented into phonemes (e.g., vowels and consonants) and that these are represented by an alphabetic orthography or written letters. This seems to be critical for the development of beginning reading skills, which—in conjunction with comprehension and other higher-level aspects—are important for advanced reading development.

RATIONALE FOR THE CURRENT TEXT

In this text, we address the major reasons for the present level of reading achievement and deafness, including the education and reading instructional practices of teachers. We are specifically interested in improving the ability of students who are deaf and hard of hearing to access print and interpret or use the information as critical readers. Much of our focus is on reading; our discussion of writing is guided by what the process of writing tells us about the process of reading (e.g., as discussed in Adams, 1990).

The information in this text is guided by three basic—albeit disputable—assumptions about reading and deafness. We will show, via research, that the English reading development of students who are deaf or hard of hearing is similar to that of students with typical hearing who are reading in English as a first language (e.g., see discussions and reviews in Hanson, 1989; Hayes & Arnold, 1992; Paul, 1998, 2003; Rose et al., 2004; Schirmer & McGough, 2005). This is true whether children and adolescents who are deaf or hard of hearing are learning to read in English as a first or as a second language. Technically, this means that the reading development of students who are deaf or hard of hearing is qualitatively similar to that of younger hearing students. That is, these students proceed through developmental stages, make errors, and use general reading strategies that are roughly similar to those of children who have typical hearing.

In essence, the view above has been labeled the *qualitative-similarity* hypothesis (Paul, 2001, 2003). This has important reading instructional implications, particularly with respect to the recommendations of the National Reading Panel (2000; see also Schirmer & McGough, 2005). It should be emphasized that this does not necessarily mean that the delivery of instruction is the same for all children, whether typical or those who are deaf or hard of hearing. Nevertheless, it does mean that certain fundamentals apply to all

children who are learning to read and write (e.g., McGuinness, 2004, 2005). For example, we know that phonics is critical for beginning reading development (e.g., National Reading Panel, 2000). Thus, all children need to be exposed to this type of instruction in order to further their understanding of phonemic awareness and to learn about the alphabetic system of English. Although phonics is important, how it is *delivered* via instruction should vary according to the individual differences in children. As an example, children who are deaf or hard of hearing who have limited or no usable residual hearing typically cannot benefit from traditional phonics instruction, but—as shown in this text—they will benefit from instruction that has been supplemented by alternative methods such as Visual Phonics (Trezek & Malmgren, 2005; Trezek & Wang, 2006; Trezek et al., 2007).

We also demonstrate that there is a strong reciprocal relationship between the conversational-based form (i.e., spoken or signed) and the written-based form (i.e., print or written language) of the same language—in this case, English (e.g., Chall, 1996; Pearson, 2004; Snowling & Hulme, 2005; Templeton & Bear, 1992). This reciprocity, our second assumption, requires that children have a working knowledge of the components of English while learning to read English. This has been supported, in part, by the strong relationship between phonemic awareness and beginning reading skills. Indeed, it has been shown that a large percentage of children who are at risk for developing beginning reading skills have phonological processing problems, particularly in the area of phonemic awareness (Adams, 1990; Pearson, 2004; Snow et al., 1998; Snowling & Hulme, 2005).

It is important to clarify the relationships among phonological awareness, phonemic awareness, and phonics that have been mentioned thus far (see also Chapters 3 & 4).

Phonological awareness is a general awareness of the sound system of a language. Children recognize that spoken language contains structures that are separate from meaning. By focusing on the internal structures of words, children can hear or recognize chunks of sounds such as syllables and rhymes. Some children are somewhat aware of smaller units of sounds such as **phonemes**; however, **phonemic awareness** (e.g., a word can be separated into phonemes such as /c/ /a/ /t/) usually develops after the general phonological awareness and typically requires instruction. One of the manifestations of phonological awareness can be seen in the way children play with words by repeating them and by the rhymes that children make up or remember (*rat-tat-tat; pitter-patter*).

Phonics is the use of instruction that assists children in understanding the systematic relations between sounds and letters—that is, letter–sound correspondences. Phonics instruction requires that children possess both phonological and phonemic awareness skills. Thus, the developmental order of progression seems to be phonological awareness, phonemic awareness, and then the use of phonics (e.g., see discussions in McGuinness, 2004; National Reading Panel, 2000; Snowling & Hulme, 2005). In essence, the use of phonics as a teaching tool is not feasible—or is extremely difficult—without a working knowledge of phonology and phonemes. Adequate development of phonemic awareness, along with vocabulary and comprehension knowledge, is necessary for the subsequent acquisition of advanced reading skills (e.g., Chall, 1996; National Reading Panel, 2000; Snow et al., 1998; Snowling & Hulme, 2005).

The third assumption guiding this text is that we believe it is necessary to teach reading skills explicitly in meaningful, structured situations. This is evident not only for struggling readers who have typical hearing, but also for many struggling readers who are deaf or hard of hearing (Paul, 1998; Rose et al., 2004; Stewart & Clarke, 2003). Typically, good readers improve their knowledge of reading, including vocabulary and concepts, by engaging in wide and varied reading activities (Stahl & Nagy, 2006). In contrast, struggling readers are not likely to be voracious, motivated readers. Thus, unlike good readers, they do not improve their reading skills in an incremental fashion by reading widely. In fact, many struggling readers do not read at all or read very little outside of the school setting (e.g., Adams, 1990, 1994; Snow et al., 1998; Stahl & Nagy, 2006). This places the teacher in a critical role with respect to reading instruction for these students. From another perspective, this means that teachers need to understand not only the process of reading, but also how to utilize and differentiate a range of instructional strategies to meet the individual needs of students who are deaf or hard of hearing.

Each of the above assumptions is addressed in detail in the remainder of this text. These assumptions support our major goal; that is, our attempt to relate the findings and principles of the National Reading Panel (2000) to teaching reading to students who are deaf or hard of hearing. It is hoped that the readers of this text will see the fallacy of current *either–or* debates (e.g., word identification or comprehension, to teach or not to teach, American Sign Language or English signing) that have polarized views on the development of reading skills with children and adolescents who are deaf or hard or hearing. The purpose of the book is to help deaf educators and other interested persons understand reading theories and research and to provide suggestions on how to adapt mainstreaming reading instructional methods (e.g., the recommendations of the National Reading Panel) into their practice.

Conclusion

Chapter 1 examined the reading difficulties of students who are deaf or hard of hearing in detail. The guiding question of the chapter was, Is reading different for deaf individuals? We conclude that the answer to this question is predominantly *no,* although we acknowledge the *yes* aspects relating to language and experience.

First, we provided a brief description of deafness. We then reported the current reading achievement and comprehension levels of students who are deaf or hard of hearing by addressing two fundamental questions: (1) How has reading achievement been measured? and (2) What do we mean by achievement? We briefly introduced the types of assessments that have been used to evaluate reading ability in children and adolescents who are deaf or hard of hearing. Furthermore, we proposed that there is a great need to research comprehension and to develop more valid reading comprehension tests for students who are deaf or hard of hearing, even though the concept of comprehension seems to be rather vague for those who hold a narrow view of reading. Next, we employed the process-and-knowledge view (Paul, 2003) as a framework for understanding the reading difficulties of students who are deaf or hard of hearing. Two reciprocal relationships were discussed: the reciprocity between the processing of print and an understanding or interpretation of the information and the reciprocity between the conversation (spoken or signed) and written forms of English. Finally, we discussed the rationale for the current text.

Chapter Summary

- The hearing loss of an individual who is deaf or hard of hearing can be categorized as slight, mild, moderate, severe, or profound. Different hearing loss might lead to different educational implications.

- Regardless of the type of test used—formal or informal—the overall reading achievement level of most deaf and many hard of hearing students seem to stabilize at the third- or fourth-grade level ceiling with an uneven growth rate from year to year.

- More research is needed to investigate what is comprehension and to develop more valid reading comprehension tests for students who are deaf or hard of hearing.

- The reciprocity between process and knowledge suggests that the process domain facilitates the better use of the knowledge domain and vice versa.

- Generally speaking, because of the reciprocal relationship that exists between the conversational (spoken or signed) and written forms of English, individuals need to learn to manipulate the conversational form of the language to facilitate the understanding of the information from the written form.

Review Questions

1. Discuss the types of assessments that have been used to evaluate reading ability in deaf or hard of hearing children and adolescents. What factor or factors have influenced these types of assessments?

2. In the chapter, it has been stated that the reading achievement level of many deaf

and several hard of hearing students seems to plateau at the third- or fourth-grade level. What are some possible reasons for this plateau?

3. Discuss the basic tenets of the following two different views in answering the question, What is reading achievement?

    (a)   A Simple View of Reading

    (b)   A broader view of reading

4. Briefly describe the reciprocal relationship between the process domain and knowledge domain in reading.

5. Briefly describe the reciprocal relationship between the conversation (spoken or signed) and written forms of English.

6. According to the authors, what are the three assumptions that guide the discussion of the information in this text?

REFLECTIVE QUESTIONS

1. Is reading different for deaf individuals? If so, why? If not, why not? Please corroborate your answer using the process-and-knowledge framework. You may also wish to use the discussion of the Hanson quote that began this chapter.

2. What are the problems associated with current reading assessments for students who are deaf or hard of hearing? What are some of the essential considerations in developing valid reading assessments for students who are deaf or hard of hearing?

3. Why is it difficult to answer the question, What is reading comprehension?

SUGGESTED READINGS AND RESOURCES

Barlett, F. (1932). *Remembering*. Cambridge: Cambridge University Press.

Bernhardt, E. (1991). *Reading development in a second language*. Norwood, NJ: Ablex.

Huey, E. (1968). *The psychology and pedagogy of reading*. New York: Macmillan. (Original work published 1908, Cambridge: MIT Press.)

Jensen, J. (Ed.). (1984). *Composing and comprehending*. Urbana, IL: National Conference on Research in English.

Kavanagh, J., & Mattingly, I. (1972). *Language by ear and by eye*. Cambridge: MIT Press.

REFERENCES

Adams, M. (1990). *Beginning to read: Thinking and learning about print*. Cambridge: MIT Press.

Adams, M. (1994). Phonics and beginning reading instruction. In F. Lehr & J. Osborn (Eds.), *Reading, language, and literacy:*

Instruction for the twenty-first century (pp. 3–23). Hillsdale, NJ: Erlbaum.

Allen, T. (1986). Patterns of academic achievement among hearing impaired students: 1974 and 1983. In A. Schildroth & M. Karchmer (Eds.), *Deaf children in America* (pp. 161–206). San Diego: Little, Brown.

Anthony, D. (1966). *Seeing essential English*. Unpublished master's thesis, Eastern Michigan University, Ypsilanti.

Babbini, B., & Quigley, S. (1970). *A study of the growth patterns in language, communication, and educational achievement in six residential schools for deaf students*. Urbana: University of Illinois, Institute for Research on Exceptional Children. (ERIC Document Reproduction Service No. ED 046 208).

Balow, B., Fulton, H., & Peploe, E. (1971). Reading comprehension skills among hearing-impaired adolescents. *Volta Review, 73*, 113–119.

Bornstein, H., Saulnier, K., & Hamiliton, L. (1983). *The comprehensive signed English dictionary*. Washington, DC: Gallaudet College Press.

Bradley-Johnson, S., & Evans, L. (1991). *Psychoeducational assessment of hearing-impaired students*. Austin, TX: Pro-Ed.

Brueggemann, B.J. (Ed.). (2004). *Literacy and deaf people: Cultural and contextual perspectives*. Washington, DC: Gallaudet University Press.

Catts, H., & Kamhi, A. (2005). *Language and reading disabilities* (2nd ed.). New York: Pearson/Allyn & Bacon.

Chall, J. S. (1996). *Stages of reading development.* (2nd ed.). New York: McGraw-Hill.

Davey, B., LaSasso, C., & Macready, G. (1983). Comparison of reading compre-hension task performance for deaf and hearing readers. *Journal of Speech and Hearing Research, 26*, 622–628.

deVilliers, P. (1991). English literacy development in deaf children: Directions for research and intervention. In J. Miller (Ed.), *Research on child language disorders: A decade of progress* (pp. 349–378). Austin, TX: Pro-Ed.

Ewoldt, C. (1987). Reading tests and the deaf reader. *Perspectives for Teachers of the Hearing Impaired, 5*, 21–24.

Farr, R., & Carey, R. (1986). *Reading: What can be measured?* (2nd ed.). Newark, DE: International Reading Association.

Fleetwood, E., & Metzger, M. (1998). *Cued language structure: An analysis of Cued American English based on linguistic principles*. Silver Spring, MD: Calliope Press

Gough, P. (1984). Word recognition. In P. D. Pearson, R. Barr, M. Kamil, & P. Mosen-thal (Eds.), *Handbook of reading research* (pp. 225–253). White Plains, NY: Long-man.

Gough, P., & Tunmer, W. (1986). Decoding, reading, and reading disability. *Remedial and Special Education, 7*, 6–10.

Gustason, G., & Zawolkow, E. (1993). *Signing exact English*. Los Alamitos, CA: Modern Signs Press.

Hanson, V. (1989). Phonology and reading: Evidence from profoundly deaf readers. In D. Shankweiler & I. Lieberman (Eds.), *Phonology and reading disability: Solving the reading puzzle* (pp. 69–89). Ann Arbor: University of Michigan Press.

Hayes, P., & Arnold, P. (1992). Is hearing-impaired children's reading delayed or different? *Journal of Research in Reading, 15*, 104–116.

King, C. (1981). *An investigation of similarities and differences in the syntactic abilities of deaf and hearing children learning English as a first or second language.* Unpublished doctoral dissertation, University of Illinois, Champaign-Urbana.

King, C., & Quigley, S. (1985). *Reading and deafness.* San Diego: College-Hill Press.

LaSasso, C. (1985). Visual matching test-taking strategies used by deaf readers. *Journal of Speech and Hearing Research, 28,* 2–7.

LaSasso, C. (1999). Test-taking skill: A missing component of deaf students' curriculum. *American Annals of the Deaf, 144* (1), 35–43.

Lipson, M., & Wixson, K. (1997). *Assessment and instruction of reading and writing disability: An interactive approach* (2nd ed.). New York: Longman.

Marschark, M. (2007). *Raising and educating a deaf child: A comprehensive guide to the choices, controversies, and decisions faced by parents and educators* (2nd ed.). New York: Oxford University Press.

McCormick, S. (1987). *Remedial and clinical reading instruction.* Columbus, OH: Merrill.

McGuinness, D. (2004). *Early reading instruction: What science really tells us about how to teach reading.* Cambridge: MIT Press.

McGuinness, D. (2005). *Language development and learning to read: The scientific study of how language development affects reading skill.* Cambridge: MIT Press.

Moores, D. (1996). *Educating the deaf: Psychology, principles, and practices* (4th ed.). Boston: Houghton-Mifflin.

Moores, D. (2001). *Educating the deaf: Psychology, principles, and practices* (5th ed.). Boston: Houghton-Mifflin.

Moores, D. (2006). Print literacy: The acquisition of reading and writing skills. In D. Moores & D. Martin (Eds.), *Deaf learners: Development in curriculum and instruction* (pp. 41–55). Washington, DC: Gallaudet University Press.

Musselman, C. (2000). How do children who can't hear learn to read an alphabetic script? A review of the literature on reading and deafness. *Journal of Deaf Studies and Deaf Education, 5,* 9–31.

National Reading Panel (2000). *Report of the National Reading Panel: Teaching children to read—An evidence-based assessment of the scientific research literature on reading and its implications for reading instruction.* Jessup, MD: National Institute for Literacy at EDPubs.

Paris, S., & Stahl, S. (Eds.). (2005). *Children's reading comprehension and assessment.* Mahwah, NJ: Erlbaum.

Paul, P. (1998). *Literacy and deafness: The development of reading, writing, and literate thought.* Needham Heights, MA: Allyn & Bacon.

Paul, P. (2001). *Language and deafness* (3rd ed.). San Diego: Singular Publishing Group

Paul, P. (2003). Processes and components of reading. In M. Marschark & P. Spencer (Eds.), *Handbook of deaf studies, language, and education* (97–109). New York: Oxford University Press.

Paul, P. (2005). Perspectives on literacy: A rose is a rose, but then again . . . maybe not. Review of Brueggemann, B. (Ed.). (2004). *Literacy and deaf people: Cultural and contextual perspectives.* Washington, DC: Gallaudet University Press. *Journal of Deaf Studies and Deaf Education, 10* (2), p. 222.

Paul, P., & Jackson, D. (1993). *Toward a psychology of deafness: Theoretical and empirical perspectives.* Needham Heights, MA: Allyn & Bacon.

Paul, P., & Quigley, S. (1990). *Education and deafness*. White Plains, NY: Longman.

Pearson, P. D. (2004). The reading wars. *Educational Policy, 18* (1), 216–252.

Pearson, P. D., & Hamm, D. (2005). The assessment of reading comprehension: A review of practices—Past, present, and future. In S. Paris & S. Stahl (Eds.). *Children's reading comprehension and assessment* (pp. 13–69). Mahwah, NJ: Erlbaum.

Pearson, P. D., & Stallman, A. (1994). Resistance, complacency, and reform in reading assessment. In F. Lehr & J. Osborn (Eds.), *Reading, language, and literacy: Instruction for the twenty-first century* (pp. 239–251). Hillsdale, NJ: Erlbaum.

Pearson, P. D., & Valencia, S. (1986, December). *Assessment, accountability, and professional prerogative*. Paper presented at the 1986 National Reading Conference, Austin, TX.

Pintner, R. (1918). The measurement of language ability and language progress of deaf children. *Volta Review, 20,* 755–764.

Pintner, R. (1927). The survey of schools for the deaf—V. *American Annals of the Deaf, 72,* 377–414.

Qi, S., & Mitchell, R. E. (2007, April). *Large-scaled academic achievement testing of deaf and hard-of-hearing students: Past, present, and future*. Paper presented at the annual meeting of the American Educational Research Association, Chicago, IL.

Quigley, S., & Paul, P. (1986). A perspective on academic achievement. In D. Luterman (Ed.), *Deafness in perspective* (pp. 55–86). San Diego: College-Hill Press.

Rose, S., McAnally, P., & Quigley, S. (2004). *Language learning practices with deaf children* (3rd ed.). Austin, TX: Pro-ed.

Ross, M. (1986). *Aural habilitation*. Austin, TX: Pro-Ed.

Russell, W., Quigley, S., & Power, D. (1976). *Linguistics and deaf children*. Washington, DC: Alexander Graham Bell Association for the Deaf.

Schirmer, B. (1994). *Language and literacy development in children who are deaf*. New York: Maxwell Macmillan International.

Schirmer, B. R., & McGough, S. M. (2005). Teaching reading to children who are deaf: Do the conclusions of the National Reading Panel apply? *Review of Educational Research, 75,* 1, 83–117.

Schow, R. & Nerbonne, M. (2007). *Introduction to audiologic rehabilitation* (5th ed.). Boston: Pearson/Allyn & Bacon.

Snow, C., Burns, S., & Griffin, P. (Eds.). (1998). *Preventing reading difficulties in young children*. Washington, DC: National Academy Press.

Snowling, M., & Hulme, C. (Eds.). (2005). *The science of reading: A handbook*. Malden, MA: Blackwell.

Stahl, S., & Nagy, W. (2006). *Teaching word meanings*. Mahwah, NJ: Erlbaum.

Stewart, D., & Clarke, B. (2003). *Literacy and your deaf child: What every parent should know*. Washington, DC: Gallaudet University Press.

Templeton, S., & Bear, D. (Eds.). (1992). *Development of orthographic knowledge and the foundations of literacy: A memorial festschrift for Edmund H. Henderson*. Hillsdale, NJ: Erlbaum.

Traxler, C. (2000). The Stanford Achievement Test, 9th edition: National norming and performance standards for deaf and hard-of-hearing students. *Journal of Deaf Studies and Deaf Education, 5,* 337–348.

Trezek, B. J., & Malmgren, K. W. (2005). The efficacy of utilizing a phonics treatment package with middle school deaf and hard-of-hearing students. *Journal of Deaf Studies and Deaf Education*, *3*, 257–271.

Trezek, B. J. & Wang, Y. (2006). Implications of utilizing a phonics-based reading curriculum with children who are deaf or hard of hearing. *Journal of Deaf Studies and Deaf Education*, *11*, 202–213.

Trezek, B. J., Wang, Y., Woods, D. G., Gampp, T. L., & Paul, P. (2007). Using Visual Phonics to supplement beginning reading instruction for students who are deaf or hard of hearing. *Journal of Deaf Studies and Deaf Education*, *12* (3), 373–384.

Trybus, R., & Karchmer, M. (1977). School achievement scores of hearing-impaired children: National data on achievement status and growth patterns. *American Annals of the Deaf*, *122*, 62–69.

Wolk, S., & Schildroth, A. (1984). Consistency of an associational strategy used on reading comprehension tests by hearing-impaired students. *Journal of Research in Reading*, *7*, 135–142.

Wrightstone, J., Aronow, M., & Moskowitz, S. (1963). Developing reading test norms for deaf children. *American Annals of the Deaf*, *108*, 311–316.

CHAPTER 2

COGNITIVE INTERACTIVE VIEW OF READING AND INSTRUCTION FOR STUDENTS WHO ARE DEAF OR HARD OF HEARING

Reading is remarkable. For some children, learning to read seems effortless and rapid, whereas for others, it can be an arduous and frustrating chore. Reading may not be rocket science, as some pundits note, but understanding how children learn to read, how to teach reading, and how to help struggling readers have been remarkably stubborn puzzles. Researchers, educators, and policy makers have devoted an enormous amount of energy and resources at the turn of this millennium to provide proven practices and evidence-based policies that will promote literacy for all children (Paris & Stahl, 2005, p. xv).

CHAPTER OBJECTIVES

After completing this chapter, the reader will be able to:

- Describe the stages of Chall's interactive theory of reading development
- Apply Chall's stage theory to the development of reading skills for students who are deaf or hard of hearing
- Explicate the finding of National Reading Panel in the five areas of instruction
- Describe the parallels between Chall's theory and the findings of the National Reading Panel

INTRODUCTION

S poken forms of languages, and probably even sign languages, have existed for almost 100,000 years (Crystal, 1997; Just & Carpenter, 1987). On the other hand, written languages are a relatively recent phenomenon, emerging about 5,000 years ago. The invention of the printing press, making printed materials more accessible and available to a wider audience, occurred about 600 years ago (Crystal, 1997; Just & Carpenter, 1987).

Despite the long historical development of reading and writing, there are ongoing debates on the answers to the following two broad questions (e.g., see McGuinness, 2004, 2005; Pearson, 2004; Snowling & Hulme, 2005): (1) What is reading? and (2) What are effective, evidence-based reading instructional strategies? The response to the first question should shed light on addressing the second one, which is probably more interesting to parents and to teachers in classroom settings. In fact, we have recently made enormous progress in understanding the nature of the reading process (National Reading Panel [NRP], 2000; Pearson, 2004). However, as the quote at the head of this chapter indicates, it has been difficult to improve the achievement of struggling readers. In other words, it has been problematic—almost a stumbling block—to figure out the nature of effective, instructional reading strategies. This is most evident for struggling readers (and writers) who are deaf or hard of hearing—the focus of this text (e.g., Antia, Reed, & Kreimeyer, 2005; Easterbrooks & Stoner, 2006; Luckner, Sebald, Cooney, Young, & Goodwin Muir, 2005/ 2006; Moores, 2006; Schirmer & McGough, 2005).

Nevertheless, it should not be surprising that the debates on the aforementioned questions are not new; they can be traced back to the 18th and 19th centuries (Bartine, 1989, 1992). Then, as now, scholars pondered over the location of meaning and how readers construct meaning. That is, scholars inquired whether meaning resided in the words on the pages of the text (similar to the earlier bottom-up models of reading; Gough, 1985). If not on the pages, perhaps, it was actually present in the reader's head (similar to the earlier top-down models of reading; Smith, 1978). Then there were those who insisted that meaning was somewhere in between, involving both the text and reader (cognitive–interactive models; Chall, 1996; Rumelhart, 1980). Still others argued that meaning was really nowhere in particular but influenced by multiple sources (transactional models; see reviews in Paul, 1998; Tierney, 1994). Apparently, it was thought that understanding the location of meaning is important for deciding how to teach readers to construct meaning or, in other words, for understanding what it is that they are reading.

Another contentious issue was the relationship between spoken English (i.e., sounds or phonemes) and its written equivalents (i.e., letters or graphemes). It was clear that written language was not simply speech being recorded by a sequence of letters on a document (e.g., McGuinness, 2004; Snowling & Hulme, 2005). On the other hand, there seemed to be a connection between the sounds of the language and the written symbols in print. Scholars wondered whether this relationship needed to be taught (i.e., via instruction) or caught (i.e., via exposure to print). Similar to the current situation, these interesting perspectives emerge from a range of scholarly disciplines including rhetoric, literary criticism, linguistics, psychology, and philosophy.

It is hoped that the readers of this text will see the fallacy of current either–or debates (e.g., word identification or comprehension; to teach or not to teach; American Sign Language or English signing) that have polarized views on the reading instruction of students who are deaf or hard or hearing. This book attempts to transform the competing forces into constructive, cooperative energy. Specifically, guided by three broad assumptions regarding reading and deafness (see the discussion in Chapter 1), our major goal of the book is to relate the findings and principles of the NRP (2000) to teaching reading to students who are deaf or hard of hearing.

*To provide a context for using the findings and recommendations of the NRP (2000), it is important to relate our framework on reading, which has been influenced mostly by **cognitive interactive views** such as Chall's model of reading development (e.g., see discussions of cognitive interactive models in Adams, 1990; Chall, 1996; McCarthey & Raphael, 1992; see also the discussion of the process-and-knowledge view in Chapter 1). Within the cognitive interactive framework, it is argued that reading is a constructive, interactive process involving the reader and the text. Although this view recognizes the contributions of the social environment, we favor the focus on the cognitive and language aspects involving the reciprocal relationship between word identification and comprehension. Chall's model fits our perception that reading is a developmental process in which reaching the advanced stage depends on—in an interactive, not linear fashion— the acquisition of fundamental skills, especially phonological and phonemic awareness and general language development (i.e., knowledge of phonology, morphology, syntax, semantics, and pragmatics). In our view, Chall's and other cognitive–interactive models are buttressed by the findings and recommendations of the National Reading Panel (2000).*

This chapter provides an introduction to Chall's stage theory of reading development. We then apply the major aspects of Chall's stage theory to the development of reading in children who are deaf or hard of hearing. The final section of the chapter details the tenets of the National Reading Panel (2000).

CHALL'S STAGES OF READING DEVELOPMENT

Probably one of the most well-known and widely accepted examples of an interactive model of reading development is the scheme developed by Jeanne Chall. Growing out of her seminal research evaluating the effectiveness of various approaches to beginning reading instruction (Chall, 1967) and coupled with her more than 25 years of experience as a clinician diagnosing and teaching individuals with severe reading disabilities, Chall presented her six-stage model of reading development in a book titled *Stages of Reading Development* (1983; 1996).

Chall (1996) hypothesized that stages of reading development resemble stages of cognitive and language development and, therefore, have a definite structure and follow a hierarchical progression. In other words, the acquisition of skills at each stage is essential to progress to the successive stages, and a failure to acquire skills at any one stage may delay or even prevent transition to the next. Children may progress through the stages at different rates in an interactive manner, but even children with special needs appear to follow the same sequence of skill development.

Chall's Stage Theory

The model that Chall (1996) proposed begins with reading readiness and ends with highly creative, complex reading. As previously stated, individuals may vary in their progression through the stages, yet most children educated in typical schools tend to progress within the age and grade limits identified. According to Chall, how well and how fast children progress through the stages depends on environmental factors, the educational opportunities provided, or both. Each of the six stages of Chall's model is briefly described in the following sections.

Stage 0: Prereading

Beginning at age six months and continuing through age six, Chall's (1996) first stage is considered a period of reading readiness and is characterized by children's growth in knowledge and use of spoken language. The acquisition of skills at this stage involves being immersed in a literate, print-rich culture and is highly dependent on interactions with adults. At this stage, children gain insights into language, syntax, and vocabulary through exposure to conversations, rhymes, alliteration, finger plays, and, most important, by being

read to by an adult. Children also begin to learn the names of the letters in the alphabet and are able to recognize words displayed in their environment. In addition, children pretend to read stories while looking at the pages of books previously read to them.

In addition to having stories read to children, activities that foster the development of skills at this stage involve interactions with adults specifically focused on the development of the skills described above. For example, while driving in the car, an adult may point out a stop sign and indicate to the child that the letters S-T-O-P mean the need to stop and wait to proceed. In subsequent car rides, the child may begin to recognize this configuration of letters and associate them with the red, octagon-shaped sign. Although the child is not technically reading the word *stop,* she is beginning to recognize that printed letters connect to meaning. If children do not obtain the skills outlined in Stage 0, then it is imperative that school programs address these critical prereading skills during Stage 1 (Chall, 1996).

Stage 1: Initial Reading and Decoding

Typically, children in Stage 1 are 6 to 7 years old and are in the first or second grade. The essential skill developed in this stage is recognizing the relation between letters and sounds and between printed and spoken words. Once children have mastered letter–sound correspondences, they are able to read simple text containing high-frequency and phonetically regular words (Chall, 1996).

To gain competency and skills in this stage, many children require direct instruction in letter–sound relations (phonics) and practice in their use. Simple stories that use words with known phonic elements and high-frequency words provide excellent independent practice. For example, the teacher may directly teach children that the letter *a* makes the sound /a/ and the letter *t* makes the sound /t/ and together these letters form the word *at*. Additional instruction can focus on adding phonemes to the beginning of *at* to form a variety of words such as *cat, hat, sat, fat, mat*, and so on. This phonetic pattern can then be reinforced and practiced while reading the book *Cat in the Hat* by Dr. Seuss both in a group and independently. In addition to children's independent reading, adults should continue to read to children not only to expose them to advanced language patterns and higher-level vocabulary, but also to increase their background knowledge. Only when children begin to concentrate on what words look like and sound like are they able to make substantial gains and progress to Stage 2 (Chall, 1996).

Stage 2: Confirmation and Fluency

Children in Chall's Stage 2 are usually 7 and 8 years old and in second and third grade. The goal of Stage 2 reading is not to gain new information but to utilize the skills acquired in the previous stages to gain automaticity and fluency with decoding and reading words. Children in Stage 2 also continue to gain new language concepts and more complex vocabulary by having stories read to them that are above their independent reading level (Chall, 1996).

To achieve automaticity and fluency, children must engage in reading of familiar, interesting materials. Teachers should provide students at this stage with short, engaging stories containing predictable patterns such as rhymes and involve them in both shared and independent reading to increase automaticity and fluency. Fluency is accomplished by integrating the knowledge of basic decoding elements, sight vocabulary, and meaning in the context of familiar stories and selections. According to Chall, adult literacy programs often fail to move readers beyond Stage 2

because the programs do not provide enough readable material containing decodable text, recognizable language, and familiar content to increase fluency. The same is true for the third-grade reader. Children who do not move beyond Stage 2 reading by the end of third grade will continue to experience difficulty and failure in school. Learning facts through reading, a major emphasis in Stage 3, will be difficult for children who have not developed adequate reading fluency (Chall, 1996).

Stage 3: Reading for Learning

Stage 3 is characterized by a shift in emphasis from learning to read to reading to learn. Chall (1996) divided Stage 3 into Phases A and B. Typically, children in Phase A are in grades four through six, whereas children in Phase B are in grades seven through nine. Reading throughout Stage 3 is used to gain new knowledge, experience new feelings, and learn new attitudes. Assuming that literacy skills are firmly developed, the focus of instruction at the beginning of fourth grade begins to shift from language arts to social studies and science. Reading skills are now being used to learn about times, places, experiences, and ideas that are removed from children's direct experience.

To acquire these skills, children read and study textbooks, reference works, chapter books, newspapers, and magazines that contain new ideas and values. Children encounter new vocabulary and syntax and must react to text through discussion, answering questions, and writing. At this stage, students should be able to apply their knowledge of decoding skills acquired and practiced in Stages 1 and 2 to effortlessly read grade-level materials. However, when students at this stage do come across an unfamiliar word, they should first attempt to decode it. If this strategy fails, they can then use their knowledge of the context to attempt to gain meaning. In the event that the meaning is still unknown, students can resort to a dictionary or thesaurus to gain meaning. Children at this stage are able to read complex fiction, biography, and nonfiction selections. As children become older and transition from Phase A to B, their ability to analyze what is being read expands and they begin to react critically to ideas. This ability to critically react to one viewpoint is prerequisite for Stage 4 reading (Chall, 1996).

Stage 4: Multiple Viewpoints

Stage 4 readers are children ages 15 to 18 who are high school sophomores, juniors, and seniors. Reading from a broad range of complex materials that are both expository and narrative in nature is characteristic at this stage. High school teachers tend to select reading materials that require children to read in greater depth and to understand a variety of viewpoints. Therefore, children at this stage must be able to simultaneously tackle layers of facts and concepts along with multiple viewpoints. For example, students at this stage may be asked to read a selection about the American Civil War and describe the reaction or perspectives of individuals in the North and the South to the expansion of slavery. Reading textbooks and studying concepts in school subjects such as science and humanities accomplish the goals of Stage 4 reading. Systematic study of vocabulary and word parts also increases the skills of children at this stage. Graduation from high school marks the end of Stage 4 and the beginning of Stage 5 (Chall, 1996).

Stage 5: Construction and Reconstruction

A Stage 5 reader is typically an adult in college. Adults at this stage read for their own purpose, and reading serves to integrate their knowl-edge with that of others. Readers at this stage are able to synthesize what they read in order to create new knowledge. Familiar materials at this stage are read at a fast pace, whereas unfamiliar material requires a slow, study-like pace. A reader at this level utilizes Stage 5 reading skills for study or work but may relax with a mystery novel that would be considered Stage 2 reading for an adult. To acquire the skills necessary to be a Stage 5 reader, adults must continue to engage in the reading of difficult material. They must be able to write papers and respond to tests and essays that call for the integration of varied knowledge and points of view (Chall, 1996).

CHALL'S STAGE MODEL AS APPLIED TO READING AND DEAFNESS

Let us further investigate the principal commonalities between Chall's stage model and the process-and-knowledge view we support and advocate (see the discussion in Chapter 1). Through this discussion, we illustrate why reading is predominately *not* different whereas some aspects of reading such as language and experience *are* different for many deaf, and some hard of hearing, individuals.

Chall's Stage Model

The reading stages described in Chall's model cannot be interpreted as static and mechanical; rather, they should be considered as continuous, overlapping, and adaptable. Furthermore, the described ages or grades at each stage are approximate (Chall, 1996). In other words, the stage model is a description of the general reading development stages with adequate room for individual differences among learners. The primary assumption of a stage model is that development at each stage depends on sufficient development at the preceding stages. The sequence of reading development should be similar for all learners, whereas different learners might progress at different rates. In the case of many deaf and some hard of hearing learners, they proceed through qualitatively similar stages as hearing learners, although they might be quantitatively delayed in the progress. The quantitative differences of these learners might relate to their unique language experiences. These qualitative similarities and quantitative differences are discussed in each stage in the following.

Stage 0: Prereading

Language is a mental tool, an actual mechanism for thinking (Vygotsky, 1962, 1978). That is, language is the carrier of social information (i.e., knowledge) as well as the tool to utilize (e.g., reflect on) the social information. At the prereading stage, the language development of children who are deaf or hard of hearing varies significantly. In extreme cases, a child with a profound hearing loss born to hearing parents who do not use a form of sign language or other meaningful communication methods at home might enter school with extremely limited language skills. It is not surprising that a deaf child without any functional language is at a disadvantage at this stage because she does not have the primary knowledge and processing skills of reading. Thus, for this child, there is a dual task: learning the language and learning to read the language.

What about children who are deaf or hard of hearing who are exposed to spoken English via the use of speech or Cued Speech/ Language, **manually coded English systems** (e.g., **signed English,** Signing Exact English),

or the combination of speech and manually coded English systems simultaneously? The quality and quantity of exposure to English varies considerably among these individuals. In addition, the degree of access to English phonology can also vary substantially. **Speech reading** alone can only provide a partial picture of spoken English (see discussion in Chapter 3). Although manually coded English systems might be effective in introducing vocabulary and syntax of English, they represent English at the morphological level—albeit incompletely—rather than at the phonemic level. Therefore, these systems might not be effective in assisting children in acquiring the beginning awareness of the sound structures of words. Even when combined, speech reading and manually coded English systems can never provide a complete picture of spoken English. Only Cued Speech/Language has the potential to sufficiently represent spoken English at the phonemic level (see also the discussion in Chapter 3).

Then what about a deaf child who is born to deaf parents who use American Sign Language (ASL) only at home? She might have the general language base to acquire necessary prior knowledge and metacognitive skills in reading, but she might still struggle with the processing (i.e., decoding, accessing print) of reading, particularly the phonological processing because of her limited exposure to and internalization of spoken English.

In a nutshell, spoken language development is critical in the prereading stage for reading English. Children need to acquire phonological information of a spoken language to obtain a beginning awareness of the sound structures of words. Of all the communication systems used by children who are deaf or hard of hearing, Cued Speech/Language seems by far the most effective method in delivering adequate phonological information of spoken

English. For students using other communication systems including speech, manually coded English systems, both speech and manually coded English systems simultaneously, or ASL only, supplementary reading instructional tools such as Visual Phonics (Cued Speech/ Language can also be used as a reading instructional tool alone) should be used to introduce the phonological information of spoken English (see further discussions in Chapters 3 and 4).

Stage 1: Initial Reading and Decoding

After children acquire the primary awareness of the sound structures of words (i.e., phonemic awareness) in Stage 0, they will proceed to Stage 1 where the instruction on the relationship between letter and sound (i.e., phonics) is emphasized. Similar to Stage 0, the various communication systems used by children who are deaf or hard of hearing might influence their acquisition of phonics skills depending on how much phonological information of spoken English these communication systems can deliver. The failure to make the connection between letter and sound might be a major underlying reason for the reading difficulties of students who are deaf or hard of hearing.

Stage 2: Confirmation and Fluency

In Stage 2, children apply their knowledge gained in Stage 1 to read words, sentences, and passages. Through practice, they can recognize most words automatically and fluently; this frees most of their cognitive attention from decoding the words. By the end of Stage 2, typically the third grade, children are generally ready to transit from *learning to read* to *reading to learn*. However, most students who are deaf or hard of hearing are unable to progress to higher stages because of the lack of

prerequisite skills from earlier stages, which might contribute to the third- or fourth-grade reading level ceiling effect previously discussed (see Chapter 1).

Stages 3–5

Unfortunately, most deaf and many hard of hearing students seem to settle at Stage 2 of the reading development and never progress to Stage 3 and above. Students who successfully progress to Stage 3 and beyond generally acquire the ability to process phonological and other information during reading, and such a skill distinguishes these skilled deaf readers from average deaf readers (see also the discussion in Chapter 3).

Conclusion on Chall's Stage Model

Chall's stage model can be used to argue that the reading development of students who are deaf or hard of hearing is qualitatively similar although quantitatively different from that of hearing peers. The major differences might be related to the communication systems they use. Through the use of ASL, it is possible for ASL–English bilingual deaf learners to develop aspects from the knowledge domain of reading such as prior knowledge and some metacognitive skills. However, some obstacles in the processing domain of reading cannot be overcome by instruction in ASL alone. These obstacles include decoding words at the phonemic level and other subsentence levels and are primarily the result of the different grammatical structures of ASL and English. Without intervention, deaf ASL users might not be able to access the phonological properties of English, which contributes to the development of decoding or word-identification skills.

With the representation of English syntax structures, manually coded English systems might be helpful in developing the processing domain of reading at the word, phrase, sentence, and passage level. Nevertheless, decoding words at the subword level (i.e., phonemic level) still poses a challenge. Speech reading can provide some information at the subword level, but the presented information is considerably insufficient and less precise. Representing phonological information of English, reading instructional tools such as Visual Phonics or Cued Speech/Language (Cued Speech/Language is also a communication system) provide promise for developing skills in the processing domain of reading for children with limited or inadequate access to sound.

Although Chall's (1996) stage theory provides a theoretical framework for understanding the importance of developing beginning reading skills and the impact of these skills on higher-level reading, her descriptions do not explicitly address instructional activities that foster the development of these skills. Therefore, to gain insight into instructional practices, the findings of the National Reading Panel (2000) are considered, especially in light of the principles of cognitive interactive models of reading.

NATIONAL READING PANEL

The NRP (2000) was established in response to a 1997 congressional directive aimed at identifying the skills and methods of instruction consistently associated with reading achievement. A panel of 14 individuals—including leading scientists in reading research, representatives of colleges of education, reading teachers, educational administrators, and parents—was charged with reviewing the vast amount of available reading research with a focus on the critical years of kindergarten through third grade.

The panel identified more than 100,000 research studies completed since 1966 and subjected them to a specific criteria for review. Relying on a carefully developed screening procedure, NRP (2000) members examined research studies that met the following criteria: (1) measured reading achievement, (2) were generalizable to the larger population, (3) compared approaches to examine their effectiveness, and (4) were deemed to be of high quality. In a field in which decisions are often based on ideology rather than scientific evidence, the rigorous criteria put forth by the NRP allowed the members to consider the evidence of effectiveness when making decisions regarding content, methods, and approaches to recommend for beginning reading instruction.

To further organize the wealth of available studies, panel members prioritized reading topics based on previous findings published by the National Research Council's Committee in *Preventing Reading Difficulties in Young Children* (Snow, Burns, & Griffin, 1998) and from information gathered through regional public hearings. In April 2000, the NRP issued a report with its findings. The panel concluded that there are five essential components of a *balanced* effective reading instruction: phonemic awareness, phonics, fluency, vocabulary, and text comprehension.

Drawing from the NRP's summary report entitled *Put Reading First—The Research Building Blocks for Teaching Children to Read Kindergarten through Grade Three* (Armbruster, Lehr, & Osborn, 2001), the following brief descriptions of the findings for each component of reading instruction are offered. In addition, the connections between the NRP's findings and Chall's stage theory are explicated for each of the five components. Subsequent chapters of this text explore in greater depth the details of the panel's findings and recommended instructional activities for the five areas of instruction for students who are deaf and hard of hearing.

Phonemic Awareness

As mentioned in Chapter 1, phonemic awareness refers to the knowledge that spoken words are composed of small units of sound called *phonemes* (see also Chapters 3 and 4). For example, the words *she* (/sh/ /e/) and *he* (/h/ /e/) each contain two phonemes, whereas the words *man* (/m/ /a/ /n/) and *rock* (/r/ /o/ /ck/) contain three phonemes. Instruction in phonemic awareness involves teaching children how to manipulate phonemes in spoken syllables and words. Children learn that words can sound the same at the beginning or end (alliteration and rhyme), that words can be broken into parts, and that the parts can be blended to form words (Armbruster et al., 2001). Chall (1996) refers to this knowledge as gaining "insights into the nature of words" (p. 13); she characterized phonemic awareness as a Stage 0 or prereading skill.

The NRP reviewed the existing data on phonemic awareness for several reasons. First, phonemic awareness has received substantial attention in recent literature (see reviews in McGuinness, 2004, 2005). Second, many studies have been conducted to explore the role that phonemic awareness plays in reading acquisition. Finally, correlational studies have found that children's knowledge of letters and phonemic awareness skills prior to entering school are the best predictors of how well they will learn to read during the first two years of instruction (Armbruster et al., 2001; McGuinness, 2004, 2005).

The panel reported strong evidence that explicit and systematic instruction in the manipulation of phonemes significantly improved students' reading skill. Moreover,

instruction in phonemic awareness was shown highly effective with a variety of learners across a range of grade and age levels. The panel concluded that phonemic awareness instruction is an essential component of reading instruction. Once children have learned to manipulate phonemes in spoken syllables and words through phonemic awareness instruction, they are prepared to benefit from instruction that focuses on the links between those phonemes and the written symbols (i.e., **graphemes**) that correspond to the phonemes (Armbruster et al., 2001; McGuinness, 2004, 2005).

Phonic Skills

Unlike phonemic awareness instruction, which deals primarily with the sounds that make up spoken words, phonics instruction deals with the linkages between spoken sounds and the corresponding written symbols. Phonics instruction therefore teaches children to link written letters to the phonemes to form letter–sound correspondences. Chall (1996) emphasized this instruction in Stage 1 and insisted that children become fluent and automatic decoders by the end of Stage 2.

The National Reading Panel concluded that phonics instruction produces significant benefits for all students in kindergarten through sixth grade and, in particular, for children who have difficulty learning to read. The evidence supporting phonics instruction, like the evidence supporting phonemic awareness instruction, is so strong that the panel recommends that it become an integral part of reading instruction. The panel also noted that systematic phonics instruction, characterized by teaching a planned sequence of phonics elements, produced the greatest improvements in reading (Armbruster et al., 2001; McGuinness, 2004, 2005). The findings of the NRP are echoed in Chall's (1996) recommendation for direct instruction of letter–sound relationships in Stage 1.

For children who have difficulty learning to read, the panel found that a combination of systematic phonics instruction and synthetic phonics instruction produced the best results compared to other approaches. Synthetic phonics instruction consists of explicitly teaching children to convert letters into sounds and to blend the sounds to form recognizable words. For all children, mastery of phonic skills progresses to reading words, sentences, and short passages. Once they begin utilizing phonic skills to read sentences and passages, children are in a position to begin to develop reading fluency (Armbruster et al., 2001; see also the discussions in McGuinness, 2004, 2005).

Fluency

According to the National Reading Panel, **fluency** is the ability to read accurately and quickly with proper expression. When reading silently, fluent readers recognize words automatically and are able to group words together in order to gain meaning from what they read. When reading orally, these same readers read as if they are speaking: effortlessly and with proper expression. In contrast, readers who are unable to read fluently read slowly, word by word, and their oral reading is considered "chopping and plodding" (Armbruster et al., 2001, p. 22).

Fluency is an important reading skill because it provides the critical bridge between word reading (i.e., word identification) and comprehension. Fluent readers, or those with automatic decoding skills, can read words effortlessly, thus freeing their cognitive energy to attend to meaning. On the other hand, less fluent readers must focus their attention on decoding the individual words; therefore, they have little energy or attention available for comprehension (Armbruster et al., 2001; see also the discussions in McGuinness, 2004, 2005). Chall (1996) also recognized the role of fluency and noted the importance of developing **automaticity** in Stage 2 through the use of familiar, decodable text.

Vocabulary

There are two types of **vocabulary**: oral vocabulary and reading vocabulary. **Oral vocabulary** refers to words we know and use in spoken language, whereas **reading vocabulary** indicates those words we recognize in print. Because beginning readers rely on words in their oral vocabulary to make sense of the words they see in print, they will have a difficult time reading words that are not part of their oral vocabulary (Note: The similarities and differences between oral vocabulary and "**sign vocabulary**" are discussed in Chapter 6 of this text.) Reading vocabulary is an important component of reading comprehension. Children must know the meaning of the majority of words in a selection in order to comprehend what they are reading (Armbruster et al., 2001; Stahl & Nagy, 2006).

Vocabulary can be learned indirectly in the context of oral communication and listening to stories being read. This type of indirect vocabulary instruction is emphasized throughout Chall's (1996) first three stages of development. However, some vocabulary must be directly taught. According to the findings of the NRP, vocabulary can best be taught through two methods: specific word instruction and word learning strategies. Specific word instruction provides students with opportunities to develop in-depth knowledge of word meanings whereas the teaching of word learning strategies enable students to use words accurately in their writing and generalize these words to spoken language (Armbruster et al., 2001; Stahl & Nagy, 2006). Chall also indicated the need for systematic word study to improve and enhance reading skills for Stage 4 readers.

Comprehension

Comprehension is the primary goal of reading; good readers have a purpose for reading and are actively engaged as they read (Paris & Stahl, 2005). This active engagement in the reading process is often referred to as **metacognition**. Metacognition can be defined as "thinking about thinking" (Armbruster et al., 2001, p. 49). Good readers employ metacognitive strategies to clarify a purpose before reading, monitor their understanding during reading, and reflect after reading. The role of metacognitive strategies is evident as the shift from learning to read to reading to learn occurs at Stage 3 of Chall's (1996) model. Throughout Stages 3 through 5, Chall emphasizes the need to analyze, synthesize, and react critically to what is read.

As with the other elements of reading, the National Reading Panel recommended explicit and direct teaching of comprehension strategies to accomplish the goal of improved and enhanced comprehension. The strategies recommended include comprehension monitoring, use of graphic and semantic organizers, answering and generating questions, recognizing story structure, and summarizing. These strategies can be taught at any age or grade level. From the earliest stages of reading, children benefit from understanding that reading is a process and that comprehension is the ultimate goal. Although some comprehension strategies may be acquired informally, explicit teaching of how and when to apply comprehension strategies is highly effective in advancing understanding (Armbruster et al., 2001; see also the discussion in Paris & Stahl, 2005).

CONCLUSIONS ON CHALL AND THE NATIONAL READING PANEL

Chall's stages provide the theoretical foundation for understanding the process of reading development, whereas the five components identified by the NRP supply the instructional activities to achieve the goals put forth in each of Chall's stages or any other cognitive–interactive model. The similarities between the two are quite evident. The importance of directly and systematically teaching children to read by third grade is emphasized by both Chall and the National Reading Panel (2000). In addition, the goals of each of Chall's stages of development parallel the findings of the panel. For example, Chall emphasized phonemic awareness activities in Stage 0; phonics was highlighted in Stage 1; fluency formed the foundation for Stage 2; indirect vocabulary development was stressed in Stages 0–3, whereas direct vocabulary instruction began at Stage 4; and text comprehension was emphasized in Stages 3 through 5 with increasing emphasis on higher-order comprehension at the more advanced stages (Carnine, Silbert, Kame'enui, & Tarver, 2004). Together, the interactive model of reading development proposed by Chall (1996) and the findings of the NRP (2000) form the framework for this text and for understanding and teaching reading to children and adolescents who are deaf or hard of hearing.

CONCLUSION

The two major intents of this chapter were (1) to provide an overview on the theoretical framework of the book—Chall's stage theory and its application for the reading instruction of students who are deaf or hard of hearing—and (2) to introduce the recommendations of the report from the National Reading Panel (2000). Our overall reading perspective is cognitive–interactive in nature and is driven by our interpretation and application of Chall's reading development model (1996). We argue that our reading perspective should be effective in offering instructional and research suggestions to improve the reading achievement levels of children and adolescents who are deaf or hard of hearing. In essence, as the evidence suggests, one of the major barriers for students who are deaf or hard of hearing is the lack of instruction regarding the phonology of English, which is the focus of the discussion in Chapter 3.

CHAPTER SUMMARY

- Chall's (1996) reading development model is one of the most well known and widely accepted examples of an interactive model of reading development. Chall hypothesized that the six stages of reading development resemble stages of cognitive and language development and therefore have

a definite structure and follow a hierarchical progression.

- The sequence of reading development should be qualitatively similar for all learners, whereas different learners, including those who are deaf or hard of hearing, might progress at quantitatively different rates. The major differences in the reading development of students who are deaf or hard of hearing might be related to the communication systems that could influence their development in the process and knowledge domains.

- The National Reading Panel (2000) proposed five essential components of a balanced effective reading instruction: phonemic awareness, phonics, fluency, vocabulary, and text comprehension.

- Chall's stages provide the theoretical foundation for understanding the process of reading development, whereas the five components identified by the NRP supply the instructional activities to achieve the goals put forth in each of Chall's stages or any other cognitive–interactive model.

REVIEW QUESTIONS

1. Briefly describe the six-stage model of reading development proposed by Chall (1996).

2. According to the report of the National Reading Panel (2000), what are the five essential components of a *balanced* effective reading instruction? Briefly describe each component.

3. Describe how the components of the National Reading Panel (2000) can be related to the stages of Chall's (1996) reading model.

4. Discuss the reciprocity of process and knowledge in the reading development of students who are deaf or hard of hearing using Chall's stage model.

REFLECTIVE QUESTIONS

1. It has been reported that average 18- to 19-year-old students with severe to profound hearing impairment are reading no better than average 9- to 10-year-old hearing students. In fact, the third- or fourth-grade reading level has been reported as a ceiling effect. This ceiling effect not only is apparent for students with severe to profound hearing impairment, but also exists for other populations including at-risk students and students in special education programs. How would you explain the existence of this ceiling effect using Chall's (1996) six-stage model of reading development?

2. "Fluency is the bridge between decoding and comprehension." Can you provide support for this statement using Chall's (1996) reading stages theory and the findings of National Reading Panel (2000)?

SUGGESTED READINGS AND RESOURCES

Baker, L., Dreher, M., & Guthrie, J. (2000). *Engaging young readers: Promoting achievement and motivation.* New York: Guilford.

Davis, F. (Ed.). (1971). *The literature of research in reading with emphasis on models.* New Brunswick, NJ: Graduate School of Education, Rutgers University.

Kintsch, W. (1974). *The representation of meaning in memory.* Hillsdale, NJ: Erlbaum.

Kozol, J. (1985). *Illiterate America.* New York: Doubleday.

Snow, C. (2002). *Reading for understanding: Toward a research and development program in reading comprehension.* Arlington, VA: RAND.

REFERENCES

Adams, M. (1990). *Beginning to read: Thinking and learning about print.* Cambridge: MIT Press.

Antia, S., Reed, S., & Kreimeyer, K. (2005). Written language of deaf and hard of hearing students in public schools. *Journal of Deaf Studies and Deaf Education, 10,* 244–255.

Armbruster, B. B., Lehr, F., & Osborn, J. (2001). *Put reading first: The research building blocks for teaching children to read kindergarten through grade three.* Jessup, MD: National Institute for Literacy.

Bartine, D. (1989). *Early English reading theory: Origins of current debates.* Columbia, SC: University of South Carolina Press.

Bartine, D. (1992). *Reading, criticism, and culture: Theory and teaching in the United States and England, 1820–1950.* Columbia, SC: University of South Carolina Press.

Carnine, D. W., Silbert, J., Kame'enui, E. J., & Tarver, S. G. (2004). *Direct instruction reading* (4th ed.). Upper Saddle River, NJ: Pearson Education.

Chall, J. S. (1967). *Learning to read: The great debate*. New York: McGraw-Hill.

Chall, J. S. (1983). *Stages of reading development*. New York: McGraw-Hill.

Chall, J. S. (1996). *Stages of reading development*. (2nd ed.). New York: McGraw-Hill.

Crystal, D. (1997). *The Cambridge encyclopedia of language* (2nd ed). New York: Cambridge University Press.

Easterbrooks, S., & Stoner, M. (2006). Using a visual tool to increase adjectives in the written language of students who are deaf or hard of hearing. *Communication Disorders Quarterly*, 27(2), 95–109.

Gough, P. (1985). One second of reading: Postscript. In H. Singer & R. Ruddell (Eds.), *Theoretical models and processes of reading* (3rd ed.) (pp. 687–688). Newark, DE: International Reading Association.

Just, M. A., & Carpenter, P. A. (1987). *The psychology of reading and language comprehension*. Boston: Allyn & Bacon.

Luckner, J. L., Sebald, A. N., Cooney, J., Young, J., & Goodwin Muir, S. (2005/2006). An examination of the evidence-based literacy research in deaf education. *American Annals of the Deaf*, 150, (5), 443–456.

McCarthey, S., & Raphael, T. (1992). Alternative research perspectives. In J. Irwin & M. Doyle (Eds.), *Reading/writing connections: Learning from research* (pp. 2–30). Newark, DE: International Reading Association.

McGuinness, D. (2004). *Early reading instruction: What science really tells us about how to teach reading*. Cambridge: MIT Press.

McGuinness, D. (2005). *Language development and learning to read: The scientific study of how language development affects reading skill*. Cambridge: MIT Press.

Moores, D. (2006). Print literacy: The acquisition of reading and writing skills. In D. Moores & D. Martin (Eds.), *Deaf learners: Development in curriculum and instruction* (pp. 41–55). Washington, DC: Gallaudet University Press.

National Reading Panel. (2000). *Report of the National Reading Panel: Teaching children to read—An evidence-based assessment of the scientific research literature on reading and its implications for reading instruction*. Jessup, MD: National Institute for Literacy at EDPubs.

Paris, S., & Stahl, S. (Eds.). (2005). *Children's reading comprehension and assessment*. Mahwah, NJ: Erlbaum.

Paul, P. (1998). *Literacy and deafness: The development of reading, writing, and literate thought*. Needham Heights, MA: Allyn & Bacon.

Pearson, P. D. (2004). The reading wars. *Educational Policy*, 18 (1), 216–252.

Rumelhart, D. (1980). Schemata: The building blocks of cognition. In R. Spiro, B. Bruce, & W. Brewer (Eds.), *Theoretical issues in reading comprehension* (pp. 33–58). Hillsdale, NJ: Erlbaum.

Schirmer, B. R., & McGough, S. M. (2005). Teaching reading to children who are deaf: Do the conclusions of the National Reading Panel apply? *Review of Educational Research*, 75(1), 83–117.

Smith, F. (1978). *Understanding reading* (Rev. ed.). New York: Holt, Rinehart, & Winston.

Snow, C. E., Burns, S. M., & Griffin, P. (Eds.). (1998). *Preventing reading difficulties in young children*. Washington, DC: National Academy Press.

Snowling, M., & Hulme, C. (Eds.). (2005). *The science of reading: A handbook*. Malden, MA: Blackwell.

Stahl, S., & Nagy, W. (2006). *Teaching word meanings*. Mahwah, NJ: Erlbaum.

Tierney, R. (1994). Dissension, tensions, the models of literacy. In R. Ruddell, M. Ruddell, & H. Singer (Eds.), *Theoretical models and processes of reading* (4th ed.) (pp. 1162–1182). Newark, DE: International Reading Association.

Vygotsky, L. (1962). *Thought and language*. Cambridge: MIT Press.

Vygotsky, L. (1978). *Mind in society: The development of higher psychological processes*. Cambridge, MA: Harvard University Press.

CHAPTER 3

PHONOLOGY AND DEAFNESS

It is critical to take note of the distinction between ASL as a visually based linguistic system and the reading of printed language as a visual process. The virtues of an effective human visual capacity transfer to sign language. They do not transfer as well to a visual process that must decode from print a spoken language. Thus, ASL is an effective language system; but visual reading of a spoken language is an incomplete language process. It must be completed by a process that refers to the writing system and the language system on which it is based. In this critical sense, then, reading is not a parallel language system. It is a process dependent on the language system. It is a process dependent on the language that provides the basis of the writing system (Perfetti & Sandak, 2000, p. 33).

CHAPTER OBJECTIVES

After completing this chapter, the reader will be able to:

- Describe the role of working memory in reading
- Explain the role of phonology in reading
- Discuss the evidence of phonological coding of deaf readers
- Identify alternative means of acquiring phonology for students who are deaf or hard of hearing
- Describe the interrelation between phonological coding, working memory, and reading achievement

INTRODUCTION

B*ecause of students' difficulty with spoken languages, there have been various arguments for the establishment of programs involving both ASL and English for students who are deaf or hard of hearing (Ewoldt, 1996; Livingston, 1997; Paul, 1990; Paul, Bernhardt, & Gramley, 1992; Reagan, 1985; Strong, 1988). The **Bilingual/Bicultural (Bi-Bi)** programs supported by the notion of a Deaf epistemology (see Chapter 1) are among them. In an educational environment influenced by Deaf epistemology, instruction is delivered through ASL, mostly in a classroom similar to what exists in residential schools, and the goal of the program is that the students are truly bilingual and bicultural. Students in these Bi-Bi programs would not only learn the common curriculum of hearing students, but also study the history of **Deaf culture** and **Deaf community**.*

Unfortunately, little empirical evidence is available on programs incorporating the use of ASL and English in bilingual situations. Most of the recently developed ASL and English programs are focused primarily on the development of written English (see review in Paul, 2001). The assumption is that it is possible to proceed from ASL to the written form of English and that the understanding or use of the primary performance form of English—that is, speech or signing—is not considered necessary. Based on their interpretations of theoretical models such as those of Cummins (1989) and Vygotsky (1962, 1978), some proponents of ASL and English bilingualism–biculturalism argue that skills acquired in one language (e.g., ASL) can be used to bypass the performance form (i.e., spoken or signed) of the target second language and still result in the ability to read and write in the second language. That is, without ever manipulating or having exposure to the performance (i.e., speech or signing) form of English print, it is still possible for deaf students to use their knowledge of ASL to acquire adequate independent English literacy skills.

Because most of the mainstream literacy models and theories are related to the students' understanding of either the phonology of English or spoken English (a performance form of English), some proponents of ASL and English bilingualism–biculturalism reject the application of mainstream literacy models and theories to deaf students. They believe that the mainstream or inclusive placements are not applicable for deaf students; they also believe that the mainstream literacy models and theories are not appropriate to address the literacy development of deaf students.

However, Paul (2001) believes that these proponents of ASL and English bilingualism–biculturalism have misinterpreted the tenets of Cummins's models (1989). Cummins's hypothesis that good readers in one language have the potential to become good readers in the second language is based on the condition that these are two spoken languages with written forms. There is little or no evidence of a correlation between proficiency in the performance mode (i.e., speech or sign) of one language and proficiency in script (i.e., reading or writing) literacy of another language, which is the case for the correlation between ASL and English print. Paul further asserts that the acquisition of adequate independent English literacy skills requires an understanding of the alphabetic principle, which in turn depends on the access to phonology and morphology of English and is facilitated by the use and understanding of the performance form of English. Paul's argument is similar to the case made in the passage by Perfetti and Sandak (2000) quoted at the beginning of this chapter.

Although we cannot change the fact that English is primarily a phonological language based on the alphabetic principle, we can utilize some modifications and adaptations of mainstream literacy models and theories to match the styles of learners who are deaf or hard of hearing. In a nutshell, mainstream literacy models and theories can and should be applied judiciously to address the literacy development of students who are deaf or hard of hearing.

Let us review what we know about reading, keeping in mind our discussion of Chall's stages of reading and the principles of the National Reading Panel in Chapter 2. The reading process is an internal semantic interpretation of visual graphemic stimuli (i.e., the print). In her landmark work, Beginning to Read: Thinking and Learning about Print, *Adams (1990) argues that "proficient reading depends on an automatic capacity to recognize frequent spelling patterns visually and to translate them phonologically" (p. 293). The role of phonology in English, or any language, is indubitable. Perfetti and Sandak (2000) claim:*

> The fundamental property of language that matches the properties of human messages is its productivity—the achievement of infinite variety in messages (semantics) by finite means from the structure of language (phonology and grammar). The phonological structure of a language provides the means to recombine meaningless sounds into basic meaning-related symbols (words and morphemes). The grammatical structure (its syntax and morphology) provides the means to recombine basic meaning-related symbols to create real messages. Systems that include structure at both levels—meaningless elements to meaningful symbols, meaningful symbols to meaningful messages—are required to provide the full range of potential human messages. (p. 33)

So what exactly is phonology? What is the role of phonology in reading? If the phonological coding superiority hypothesis in reading is valid—that is, individuals who fail to process print phonologically will generally find it difficult to become successful readers—then what are some alternative means of acquiring phonology for students with limited or inadequate access to phonology such as students who are deaf or hard of hearing?

The plan for this chapter is as follows. To highlight the importance of phonology during reading, we need to discuss, initially, the contributions of working memory to the development of reading and then provide additional information on the role of phonology during reading. Next, we will synthesize the research on the use of a phonological code during reading or reading-related tasks by students who are deaf or hard of hearing. Finally, we will describe the use of alternative mechanisms to develop phonology. It should be clear by the end of this chapter that there are strong interrelations among phonological coding, working memory, and reading achievement.

WORKING MEMORY AND READING

Working memory, also called *short-term memory*, refers to a limited-capacity mental system responsible for the temporary storage and processing of information necessary to handle tasks that require comprehension, learning, and reasoning (Baddeley, 1990). Working memory is a storage and processing system for modality-specific information. For more details on the structure of working memory, readers should consult the work of Baddeley (1986).

Research studies with both hearing and deaf students support the view that working memory is responsible for simultaneously retaining information that has just been read as well as processing previously read information (see reviews in LaSasso & Metzger, 1998; Snowling & Hulme, 2005). However, working memory during reading must be divided between processing and storage demands because of the limited capacity:

> When processing demands, such as word recognition, are excessive (as they are likely to be for younger or less-skilled readers), storage capacity is reduced. Readers with inefficient processing abilities, whether related to phonological recoding, syntactic processing, or other processing abilities, suffer from reduced working memory capacity as more energy is devoted to the processing of information, such as word identification.
>
> (LaSasso & Metzger, 1998, p. 270)

LaSasso and Metzger (1998) use the following sentence to demonstrate the significance of working memory during reading: "Mr. Green's big, white, colonial house, on the grassy knoll, behind Maple Street, was recently demolished by a bulldozer" (p. 270). By the end of the sentence, an unskilled reader without a proper usage of the working memory might lose the main message in the sentence—that is, the house was demolished. Furthermore, research studies with typical hearing students support the strong relationship between phonological working memory span and vocabulary size (Gathercole & Baddeley, 1989, 1990; see also the review in Snowling & Hulme, 2005).

Miller (1956) conducted a seminal study to measure the capacity of working memory and suggested that the typical capacity of working memory is approximately 7 ± 2 items. There has been a steady finding in the research (see the review in Hanson, 1991) that, measured by materials in print or signs, the verbal memory span of deaf individuals is shorter than that standard capacity. Even the average working memory of a deaf ASL user, although sufficient for using ASL, is only about 5 ± 1. Furthermore, the reported shorter memory span appears to be related to cognitive processes involved in short-term memory for linguistic materials only, not for nonverbal stimuli. Although Boutla and colleagues (Boutla, Supalla, Newport, & Bavelier, 2004) claimed that the 7 ± 2 memory span was an exception in spoken language, in the field of reading it is commonly accepted that, for deaf individuals, the inability to fully access spoken language "has the important consequence of limiting the development and the efficiency of phonological coding, which has consequences for the verbal short-term memory processes that underlie reading" (Hanson, 1991, p. 160).

In essence, working memory plays a critical role for storing and processing information during reading. With respect to Baddeley's (1986) model, phonological processing is able to enhance the capacity of working memory. However, it has been heavily debated on the manner in which deaf readers cognitively code printed words in their working memory. Five types of internal coding strategies are used by deaf individuals: sign, dactylic (i.e., finger spelling), phonological based, visual (i.e., orthographic), and multiple (i.e., the combinations of the above) (see the review in Paul, 2001). Nevertheless, as is documented later, the bulk of the evidence reveals that individuals who are deaf or hard of hearing who use predominantly a phonological code in working memory tend to be better readers than the individuals who predominantly use a non-phonological code. One critical issue is the ability of these individuals to use a phonological code adequately. This idea is discussed later in the use of alternative techniques for developing phonology. First, we need to provide additional information on phonology and then discuss further the relationship of phonology to the development of reading.

PHONOLOGY AND READING

In spoken languages, the term *phonology* refers to the sound structure of speech. Particularly, it is related to the perception, representation, and production of speech sounds. Thus, the phonological aspects of language include its prosodic dimensions (e.g., intonation, stress, and timing) and its articulatory units (e.g., words, syllables, and phonemes) (Snow, Burns, & Griffin, 1998). Although the term *phonology* is often associated with acoustic or auditory (sound), the phonological units of a language are not sounds. Instead, phonological units are linguistically defined primitives related to articulatory gestures. Thinking of phonological units as cognitive units rather than as sounds is essential to understanding how students who are deaf or hard of hearing can acquire knowledge of phonology and apply it to beginning reading tasks. Furthermore, phonology does not pertain only to spoken languages. For example, phonology in ASL means linguistic primitives related to the visible gestures articulated by the hands, face, and body of the signer (Hanson, 1991). However, in this text, we use phonology to refer to the phonology of spoken English.

In English, as in any other alphabetic language, the printed symbols—that is, letters or graphemes—systematically represent the component sounds of the language (Adams, 1990; Snow et al., 1998). The development of reading skills entails matching the phonemes (sounds) to the graphemes (letters) of English. Reading is "training the eye to do the work of the ear" (Moores, 2006, p. 43). Decoding print should involve learning phoneme or grapheme (sound or letter) correspondence, or phonics, provided that the child has proficiently developed skills in phonology, **morphology, syntax,** vocabulary, and **pragmatics** (Moores, 2006).

The awareness that words are composed of letters that are related to phonemic segments (e.g., phonemes) from spoken language—in other words, the awareness that written spellings systematically represent spoken words—is referred as *the knowledge of alphabetic principle*. The difficulty in understanding and using the alphabetic principle at the onset of reading acquisition is considered as the first potential stumbling block that is "known to throw children off course on the journey to skilled reading" (Snow et al., 1998, p. 4). It is not surprising that students who are deaf or hard of hearing are at risk for not acquiring sufficient knowledge of the alphabetic principle to access print because of the limited access to and instruction focused on the phonological aspects of the English language.

As discussed in Chapter 2, this text adopts the interactive cognitive-processing model as an avenue to understanding the reading process (e.g., Adams, 1990, 2004; Chall, 1996). According to Adams (1990) and others (see discussion in Tierney, 1994), the reading process involves a circular connection of four processors—**orthographic,** phonological, meaning, and context—that operate in tandem during reading. Direct visual processing (i.e., orthographic processing) and phonological translation occur simultaneously in skillful word recognition. Meaning has to be attached to the identified word at the same time to make sense of the word. Concurrently, information from the context speeds up the reader's ability to comprehend the word. Thus, orthographic, phonological, meaning, and contextual processing harmoniously occur at the same time during reading. We want to emphasize that skillful reading can only happen when all four processors are engaged cooperatively and interactively; however, our focus here is on discussing the importance of the phonological processor.

Phonological Processing

Both the orthographic and phonological processors can accept information from the outside: print information for the orthographic processor and speech information for the phonological processor. Nevertheless, only the orthographic processor is able to receive information directly from the print. Then, other than reading aloud from the print, what is the function of the phonological processor?

Adams (1990) summarizes the importance of phonological processing during reading as follows:

> For the skillful reader, automatic phonological encoding subserves two distinct and critical processes. First, as an alphabetic backup system, it increases the speed and completeness with which the meanings and orthography of less familiar words can be processed. Second, through the "articulatory loop," it expands the reader's verbatim memory capacity in support of proper comprehension. (pp. 190–191)

In other words, after a reader encounters a meaningful word multiple times, the orthographic processor instantly handles the orthographic pattern as a whole; simultaneously, the word's meaning and phonological image is stimulated. However, in the case of less familiar words, the phonological processor plays the important role of an alphabetic backup system because the units of the phonological processing (phonemes) are the building blocks of the language.

In short, phonological processing plays an essential role in reading. Meanwhile, orthographic, phonological, meaning, and contextual processors need to be working on the same thing at the same time to effectively coordinate and facilitate each other. That is, orthographic, phonological, semantic, and contextual analysis of the print word should occur simultaneously during reading.

PHONOLOGICAL CODING OF DEAF READERS

It has been widely recognized that phonology plays a vital role in enhancing word-identification skills among hearing readers (see the review in Adams, 1990; National Reading Panel, 2000; Snow et al., 1998); however, the capability of deaf readers to use phonology effectively in word identification has yet to be confidently established. This section reviews the literature on whether phonologically based coding strategies have been used effectively by deaf readers. If this is the case, then we ask the question of whether the use of phonological coding is correlated with reading proficiency in deaf readers. We then explore alterative coding mechanisms. Finally, facing the increasing cases of cochlear implants, we investigate the promise of cochlear implantation in acquiring phonology.

Evidence on Phonological Coding and Its Relationship to Reading Proficiency

There have been several comprehensive reviews of the literature on the phonological coding of readers who are deaf or hard of hearing (Alegria, 1998; Hanson, 1991; Marschark & Harris, 1996; Perfetti & Sandak, 2000). Our review here is selective, focused on representative experimental research that provided evidence that did or did not support phonological coding of deaf readers or discussed the relationship between phonological coding and reading proficiency for deaf readers.

Conrad's (1979) seminal work validated the use of phonological coding in deaf readers. Using words that sound similar but look different and words that look similar but sound different, he explored whether deaf participants who were 15 or 16 years old used *internal speech* (i.e., phonological-based codes) or visual (i.e., orthographic) codes in word identification. He found that "degree of deafness in itself is not a major factor in reading comprehension. What seems to be much more important, apart from intelligence, is whether or not the child has acquired the use of internal speech. Internal speech shows as a highly confounding factor in reading performance, as it does in short-term memory" (Conrad, 1979, p. 157).

Kelly (1993) investigated whether deaf readers use phonological coding in recalling function words and inflections. As a part of this experiment, high school deaf students were asked to determine whether strings of letters that were either phonologically and orthographically similar or only orthographically similar constituted real English words. Results indicated that participants had a faster reaction time for word pairs that were phonologically and orthographically similar; this revealed that

deaf readers' had access to phonological information. Furthermore, the skilled deaf readers showed better ability to access phonological information than did the average deaf readers.

In a recent study, Colin and colleagues (Colin, Magnan, Ecalle, & Leybaert, 2007) assessed deaf prereaders and hearing peers on measurements of rhyme decision and generation tasks in French. The results not only provided the evidence for acquiring phonological skills in deaf children, but also showed that for both hearing and deaf participants, the phonological skills acquired before learning to read predicted the written word recognition score after one year of reading instruction.

Hanson and her colleagues conducted a series of research studies on the different coding strategies of readers with profound hearing loss and unintelligible speech for whom ASL was their first language. For example, they compared the use of speech (i.e., phonological) coding and finger spelling coding for deaf beginning readers (Hanson, Liberman, & Shankweiler, 1984), the use of phonological coding and orthographical coding for deaf college students and hearing college students (Hanson & Wilkenfeld, 1985), and the use of phonological coding and sign coding for college deaf students who used ASL and hearing college students (Hanson, Goodell, & Perfetti, 1991). The findings confirmed that, similar to their hearing peers, many deaf readers learned to utilize phonological coding in word identification.

The Belgian team of Leybaert, Alegria, Charlier, and Lechat (Alegria, Charlier & Mattys, 1999; Alegria & Lechat, 2005; Charlier & Leybaert, 2000; Leybaert, 1998, 2000; Leybaert & Charlier, 1996; Leybaert & Lechat, 2001a) have also conducted series of research investigations not only to document the phonological processing of deaf children, but also to introduce Cued Speech (or Cued Speech/

Language) as a means of delivering complete phonological information to deaf individuals. For example, Leybaert (2000) engaged three groups of students who were matched for general spelling level: (1) hearing students, (2) deaf students exposed to Cued Speech early and intensely at home (CS-Home), and (3) deaf students exposed to Cued Speech later and at school only (CS-School). Results indicated that most of the spelling productions of the hearing participants as well as the CS-home participants were phonologically accurate (i.e., phonological substitutions, misspellings with pronunciations that are identical to those of the targets, e.g., SITRON for *citron*) whereas CS-school participants who had less specified phonological representations produced less phonologically accurate spellings. The researcher concluded that the acquisition of orthographic representations with high precision depends on fully specified phonological representations. We discuss the Cued Speech system further in a later section of this chapter.

An international team of LaSasso, Crain, and Leybaert (2003) compared the rhyme-generation ability of three groups of students: (1) hearing students, ages 19–21; (2) prelingually severe to profound deaf students with Cued Speech background, ages 16–24; and (3) prelingually severe to profound deaf students without Cued Speech background, ages 17–26. Correct rhyming responses were classified as being either orthographically similar (O-S) (e.g., *glue* for the target *blue*) or orthographically different (O-D) (e.g., *fare* for the target *bear*). The results indicated that the hearing participants and deaf students with a Cued Speech background relied more on phonology whereas the deaf students without a Cued Speech background relied more heavily on spelling to generate rhyme. The implication of the study was that deaf readers could use Cued Speech to develop phonological abilities.

Several other studies have also compared deaf students with their hearing peers with respect to sensitivity to phonology and spelling strategies (e.g., Johnson, Padak, & Barton, 1994; Sutcliffe, Dowker, & Campbell, 1999). The general findings indicated that the spelling strategies of deaf students were phonologically similar to those of hearing students, although their strategies requiring phonological awareness were limited. Dyer and colleagues (Dyer, MacSweeney, Szczerbinski, Green, & Campbell, 2003) studied deaf students and hearing students in the United Kingdom to investigate two cognitive factors that are typically correlated with reading delay in hearing students: Phonological Awareness and Decoding (PAD) and Rapid Automated Naming (RAN) of visual materials, which refers to the ability to name (by speech or signing) a sequence of written or pictured items quickly. The results indicated that PAD showed a relationship with reading achievement as measured by the National Foundation for Educational Research Group Reading Test (NFER-GRT) in both hearing and deaf students, whereas RAN seemed not.

Luetke-Stahlman and Nielsen (2003) explored the correlation of phonemic awareness, English language knowledge, and reading ability among deaf students. Two groups of students were compared in the study: one group with students who had been exposed to Signing Exact English (SEE II, a signing system in which a sign represents each morpheme of a word) for 5 or more years and another group with students who had been exposed to SEE for less than 2 years. Reading ability was measured through a passage-comprehension task whereas phonemic awareness was measured through a task requiring participants to substitute one phoneme for another to create new words. Participants in the longer exposure group outperformed their counterparts on all measures. Results also indicated that students with the higher reading ability also were more able to (1) provide synonyms (e.g., big–little), antonyms (e.g., hot–cold), and analogies of reading words and phrases; (2) read more listed words; and (3) use phonemic awareness skills.

On the contrary, there have been relatively few studies that provide a different perspective on the coding strategies of deaf children and adolescents. For example, Izzo's (2002) research challenged the correlation between phonemic awareness and reading ability. Elementary students who had prelingually severe to profound hearing loss participated in this study. Reading ability was measured by a retelling task, and phonemic awareness was measured by a word-to-word matching task. The results indicated that although higher scores on the reading ability task correlated with higher scores on the language ability task, no such relationship between the reading ability task and the phonemic awareness task was found.

Miller (2002) suggested that there is a causal link between phonological coding and the modal nature of a reader's primary language. Three groups of participants from Israel were included in this study: (1) prelingually deaf students raised by hearing parents who communicated orally both at home and at school, (2) prelingually deaf students whose preferred means of communication was Israeli Sign Language and most of whom were children of deaf parents, and (3) hearing students. In Hebrew, a significant part of the vowel information is represented by means of small diacritical marks (dashes and points) instead of by letter graphemes inserted between consonantal letters. Furthermore, the diacritics in Hebrew are optional. Results showed that, for both the hearing participants and the oral deaf students, the addition of vowel diacritics interfered with task performance only when it affected the target nouns'

phonological form. However, for the signer participants, the effect of three pointed stimuli categories was essentially the same. Therefore, the author concluded that the hearing and oral deaf participants visually presented the target words phonologically; however, such a pattern did not appear in the participants who were native signers.

In another study (Miller, 2004), elementary school students with prelingual deafness and control hearing students in Israel were exposed to eight experimental conditions (i.e., eight flash cards); four used written Hebrew stimuli and four used drawn stimuli. The phonological information in these stimuli was manipulated to assess the participants' processing strategies. The results of the study showed that both groups of participants showed similar information-processing skills no matter what stimuli (i.e., words or drawings) they were exposed to or whether the referencing of conceptual knowledge was required in the processing. Miller (2004) concluded that both groups used similar processing strategies for the stimuli but neither used a phonology-based strategy.

In essence, although a few studies have specifically documented the limited phonological processing of students who are deaf or hard of hearing, substantial research has suggested that deaf readers, particularly more skilled readers, have access to phonological information. Even though deaf readers' phonological coding skills are generally lower or less efficient than those of their hearing counterparts, their phonological awareness development follows the same sequence of skill development as that for hearing readers. Furthermore, there is growing concurrence that not only does phonology play an essential role in reading comprehension, but also that the ability to process phonological information during reading distinguishes skilled deaf readers from average deaf readers:

Much of this research is predicated on the theory that phonological coding is most efficiently stored in working memory. To comprehend text, working memory must be able to hold several words long enough to process complete sentences. If the reader is using a coding strategy that puts so much demand on working memory that few words can be retained while processing the meaning of a sentence, then comprehension will suffer.
(Schirmer & Williams, 2003, p. 114)

In fact, Leybaert (1993) suggested that the failure to appropriately address the phonological components of reading instruction for deaf individuals directly causes their reading problems. In Schirmer and McGough's (2005) comprehensive review of reading instruction for students who are deaf or hard of hearing, they indicated, "It is noteworthy that the researchers do not consider the probability that many of the deaf participants in these studies were taught to attend to phonological features of words through phonemic awareness activities, auditory discrimination activities, or phonic analysis instruction, and that differences in capabilities may be accounted for by differences in instruction" (p. 89).

Alterative Coding Mechanisms for Deaf Readers

Phonology of English is accessible to hearing children through the auditory channel and via the medium of speech. For obvious reasons, the auditory signal is absent or unreliable for children who are deaf or hard of hearing, and, consequently, the accessibility of phonology is denied or limited. This leads to the question of whether or not we can develop alternative coding mechanisms such as visual or sign to enhance reading instruction for this population of students.

In order to visually represent the structure of English (e.g., English words and word parts), and to assist parents in learning and using signing without learning a new language, manually coded English systems such as the **Rochester method**, Seeing Essential English (SEE I), Signing Exact English (SEE II), **Conceptually Accurate Sign English (CASE)**, signed English (SE), **Pidgin Sign English (PSE)** and **contact signing** (see the review in Paul, 2001) were developed. These signed systems are morphologically based systems for representing English morphemes although the representation of morphology is not complete. **Morphemes** are the smallest units of speech that carry meaning. For example, the word *cats* contains two morphemes: /cat/ and /s/. As building blocks of a language, phonemes are combined to form morphemes and morphemes are combined to form words or phrases. Unfortunately, manually coded English systems do not convey phonemic information (i.e., vowels and consonants) about English; rather, these signed approximations of English convey English deficiently at the morphological and syntactic levels (Kyllo, 2003; LaSasso & Crain, 2003; LaSasso & Metzger, 1998).

The reading process for students using manually coded English systems is a game of matching the sight words to signs in their sign vocabulary. Making it even more difficult, the sight words are from a language of only minimal or fractional knowledge for learners who are deaf or hard of hearing. Thus, these learners are learning to read English in print and learning the language of English concurrently. Compared to their hearing peers, deaf learners need more cognitive power during the reading process to compensate for their imperfectly developed grammatical skills and a limited vocabulary bank. The reading problems of deaf learners are correlated with the difficulties in their language processes underlying reading (Kyllo, 2003; Moores, 2006).

Promise of Cochlear Implantation in Acquiring Phonology

Since the U.S. Food and Drug Administration's November 1984 formal approval, 11.2% of children and youth who are deaf and hard of hearing in the United States have had a **cochlear implant** (Gallaudet Research Institute, 2005). When coupled with postimplantation therapy, cochlear implants can give a person who is deaf a useful auditory understanding of the environment and help him understand speech. Accruing evidence has shown improved language and speech skills (i.e., speech perception skills, speech production abilities, and oral language development) for children with cochlear implantation (e.g., Cheng, Grant, & Niparko, 1999; Geers, Nicholas, & Sedey, 2003; Miyamoto, Svirsky, & Robbins, 1997; Tomblin, Spencer, Flock, Tyler & Gantz, 1999; Tye-Murray, Spencer, & Woodworth, 1995). It seems that cochlear implants can facilitate the development of functional language and speech skills for children. Whether the communication gains are sufficient to contribute to the improvement of literacy skills is still under question.

Currently, research on the literacy skills of children with cochlear implants is emerging (see the review in Marschark, Rhoten, & Fabich, 2007). Several studies have focused on the multiple factors that affect the development of reading skills for cochlear implant users (Connor & Zwolan, 2004; Geers, 2002, 2003, 2004). A few research studies have also focused on comparing the language and literacy outcomes of children using cochlear implants with their hearing peers or other deaf children who have not received cochlear implants (Fagan, Pisoni, Horn, & Dillon, 2007; Moog, 2002; Spencer, Barker & Tomblin, 2003; Spencer, Tomblin, & Gantz, 1997;

Vermeulen, van Bon, Schreuder, Knoors, & Snik, 2007). In addition, two investigations have assessed the phonological processing skills of children using cochlear implants: Houston, Carter, Pisoni, Kirk, and Ying (2005) and Willstedt-Svensson, Lofqvist, Almqvist, and Sahlen (2004). Although both studies found evidence of phonological coding in children using cochlear implants, they also reported the impaired (i.e., inadequate use of) phonological processing skills of these children.

Overall, as revealed in the Marschark Rhoten, and Fabich (2007) review, although the positive effects of cochlear implantation on reading and academic achievement in young deaf children are apparent, empirical evidence has been inconsistent or equivocal to some degree. More methodologically strong empirical research studies as well as theoretical studies are needed in this area.

In sum, the general research findings suggest that deaf readers also use phonological coding during reading and that the phonological development of deaf readers is qualitatively similar albeit quantitatively delayed when compared with that of hearing readers. Because the manually coded English systems represent spoken English at the morphemic level (although incompletely) instead of at the phonemic level, which is the building block of English, these systems do not contain any phonological information. Consequently, these English sign systems do not provide effective coding mechanisms for deaf readers. Even though cochlear implants provide many deaf children with access to sound and an auditory-based language, such access varies significantly among individuals. It is naïve to assume that children with cochlear implants proficiently encode the phonological representations of spoken words and map phonological representations onto meanings naturally. Most children who are deaf or hard of hearing, including many children with cochlear implants, need some alternative, supportive means of acquiring phonology.

ALTERNATIVE MEANS OF ACQUIRING PHONOLOGY

It is undeniable that deaf children's lack of complete access to the auditory aspects of English puts them at a disadvantage for establishing a phonological representation (i.e., cognitively) through speech. Fortunately, there are other alternatives available to assist deaf readers in developing a phonological code. For example, visual information from speech reading and gestural information from speaking might offer deaf individuals some access to phonological information in spoken language. However, the question remains whether or not individuals who are deaf or hard of hearing can build useful phonological representations of the print words in the absence of complete auditory access to spoken English. Four major alternative means for facilitating the acquisition of phonology are discussed here: speech reading, articulatory feedback, Cued Speech (or Cued Speech/ Language) and Visual Phonics.

Speech Reading

Speech reading, previously referred to as *lip reading*, refers to the process of understanding a spoken message through observation of the speaker's face (Paul, 2001). Studies of speech reading have demonstrated equal or better ability of speech reading among hearing individuals compared to deaf individuals trained in speech reading, indicating a possible visual component in the phonological coding of hearing individuals (see the review in Hanson,

1991). In addition, the famous *McGurk effect* (McGurk & MacDonald, 1976) described a phenomenon that, when facing mismatched auditory and visual information, the actual phoneme perceived by hearing individuals is a combination of both the visual information they see from the lips of the speaker and the auditory information they actually hear. For example, when hearing participants were shown a face pronouncing the syllable /gah/ with a simultaneously auditorily presented /bah/, they perceived /dah/. This evidence supports the hypothesis that the development of phonological system through speech may be bimodal—that is, an audio channel from speech and a visual channel from speech reading. Consequently, the visual dimension of the phonological code might enable deaf readers to access the same phonological information visually.

Speech reading indisputably contributes to the development of phonological representations in deaf individuals. Furthermore, extensive research supports its role in speech perception process for both deaf and hearing individuals (see the review in Alegria et al., 1999). However, speech reading can provide only partial phonological information. That is, lip movements can provide clues about place of articulation, but nothing related to nasality or voicing. For example, via visual information on the lips alone, one cannot discriminate consonants produced at the same articulation point (e.g. /b/, /p/, and /m/). Thus, compared to the phonological information based on auditory input for hearing individuals, the phonological information captured in visual speech reading is dramatically insufficient and less precise. In fact, although orally educated deaf children have been reported to develop some phonological representations through speech reading, these representations are generally too incomplete to support efficient cognitive processing (see the review in Charlier & Leybaert, 2000).

Articulatory Feedback

Several authors have argued that the acquisition of phonological information by individuals who are deaf or hard of hearing relies on the combination of sources such as speech reading and **articulatory feedback** rather than simply one source (Leybaert, 1993). LaSasso (1996) used the term *tactile-kinesthetic* feedback system to describe how articulatory feedback can assist deaf readers in gaining phonological information about print. The **tactile-kinesthetic feedback system** refers to mouth movements combined with vocal sensations (e.g. voiced, unvoiced, etc.) that are produced to represent each phoneme. Using the example provided above of the three consonants produced at the same articulation point, /b/, /p/, and /m/, a voiced response would accompany the /b/ sound, an unvoiced response associated with the /p/ and a nasal sound would be produced to represent the /m/.

It is hypothesized that this tactile-kinesthetic feedback system functions similarly to the auditory feedback system used by hearing readers. Using this system, LaSasso (1996) suggested that a student who is deaf or hard of hearing uses the knowledge of how a phoneme or a series of phonemes feels on the mouth and in the vocal tract to determine the resulting grapheme or word. When encountering words in print, hearing readers use auditory feedback to review possible pronunciations of the word. In the same manner, readers who are deaf or hard of hearing can use the tactile-kinesthetic system feedback to review possible *pronunciations* of the word. This system may also allow visual information to be coded into phonological information.

It is of interest that this tactile-kinesthetic feedback system does not appear to be depen-dent on the students' ability to verbally pronounce the resulting word accurately. However, it is dependent on the consistent use of the appropriate mouth movement and vocal sensation to represent each phoneme. Children who are deaf or hard of hearing are likely to recognize the word if the series of phonemes is similar to one previously produced. There appears to be some promise in using this tactile-kinesthetic feedback system with students who are willing and able to produce vocal sensations. For those students who are incapable or unwilling, another alternative must be sought (see the discussion of Cued Speech and Visual Phonics included in this chapter).

Cued Speech

Cued Speech (or Cued Speech/Language) is a sound-based, visual communication system that uses eight handshapes in four different locations in combination with the natural mouth movements of speech. During cuing, the speaker keeps his hand near his mouth while speaking. Thus, speech reading is completed by the adding discriminating information (i.e., the manual gestures or cues). The emphasis is on visually representing the sounds of spoken language—that is, delivering complete phonological information. Cued Speech was initially developed to help deaf children decode speech by eliminating speech reading ambiguities so that it could further assist their language and literacy development in English (Cornett, 1967). It has now been adapted to more than 56 languages (Cornett & Daisey, 1992). Cued Speech is neither a language nor a philosophy; it is a communication system.

In Cued Speech, sets of consonants are represented by handshapes, whereas sets of vowels are represented by hand positions and sometimes hand positions plus movements (see the example for cuing the long vowel /o/ below). The general rule is that visually undistinguishable phonemes are represented by different handshapes or positions. For example, /b/ is represented by Handshape 4 (index finger, middle finger, ring finger, and little finger), /p/ is represented by Handshape 1 (index finger only), and /m/ is represented by Handshape 5 (all fingers). Within each set, phonemes are easily distinguishable through speech reading. For example, Handshape 3 (middle finger, ring finger, and little finger) represents consonants /h/, /s/, and /r / whereas the position at the mouth represents vowels /ee/ as in *see* and /er/ as in *her*. To cue the word *see*, you would hold up three fingers (middle finger, ring finger, and little finger) and put them on your mouth. Thus, one gesture completely represents this single-syllable word that consists of both a consonant and a vowel. In other words, Cued Speech represents speech at the syllable level.

For instructional purposes, Cued Speech can also be used at the phoneme level. For instance, if you want to cue a consonant alone, you hold the handshape and put it on the side of your face. To cue /p/, for example, you hold up your index finger as in Handshape 1 and put it on the side of your face. On the other hand, if you want to cue a vowel alone, you hold Handshape 5 and put it in the corresponding position. To cue the long vowel /o/ as in *bone*, you put all your fingers as in Handshape 5 on the side of your face and move forward (for further details, including pictorial representations, please see Fleetwood & Metzger, 1998).

The purpose of developing this communication system was to improve the early English language development of children who are deaf or hard of hearing and to provide them with a foundation for English reading and writing (Alegria et al., 1999). The underlying

hypothesis of Cued Speech is that, through a visual channel rather than an auditory channel, a prelingually deaf child could acquire spoken language in a way that is similar to that of a hearing child if the phonetic components of speech are represented visually (i.e., a combination of mouth movements, finger configurations, and placements of the hand).

LaSasso and colleagues (LaSasso & Crain, 2003; LaSasso & Metzger, 1998) systematically reviewed the research on Cued Speech and on the manually coded English systems. As discussed previously, manually coded English systems do not convey phonological information of English; however, Cued Speech does convey a more complete picture of spoken English at the phonemic level. Furthermore, when compared to manually coded English systems, Cued Speech requires less memory by its users to become fluent. In fact, it is reported that the system can be acquired in two days; with practice, many users can become fluent in six weeks to a few months. In addition, Cued Speech demands less cognitive processing energy because it entails coding a language (i.e., transliterating) rather than translating it as is the case with sign English. LaSasso and Crain (2003) provided an example: "[T]he shoe-fly beetle was eaten by the blue jay" (p. 33). The signer needs to decide which signs to use to represent *shoe-fly beetle* (BUG) and *blue jay* (BLUE + BIRD) or whether finger spelling should be used. It can be seen from this example that the process of translation involves a heavier mental burden than the process of transliteration required when using Cued Speech.

There is research evidence supporting the use of Cued Speech to improve speech processing for students who are deaf or hard of hearing (Alegria et al., 1999; Clarke & Ling, 1976; Leybaert, Alegria, Hage, & Charlier, 1998; Ling & Clarke, 1975; Nicholls & Ling,

1982; Vieu et al., 1998). Improved speech processing has been reported to assist students who are deaf or hard of hearing in tasks involving phonological processing such as rhyme judgments (Charlier & Leybaert, 2000), rhyme generation (LaSasso, Crain, & Leybaert, 2003), and spelling (Leybaert, 2000, Leybaert & Lechat, 2001b), as well as a set of cognitive skills involving rhyming, remembering, and reading (Leybaert & Charlier, 1996).

Cued Speech has been used with students with hearing losses, symptoms of autism, Down syndrome, deaf-blindness, cerebral palsy, and auditory processing deficits. It has also been used by general education teachers for phonics instruction and speech therapists for articulation therapy (National Cued Speech Association, 2007).

Although the Cued Speech system is 40 years old, it has not been widely used with children who are deaf or hard of hearing partially because the name Cued Speech gives the false impression that the system was designed for speech development only. Furthermore, supporting theory and research for Cued Speech has not been available until recently. Moores (1969) raised the question of interindividual and intraindividual consistency in Cued Speech and warned about the further complication of the existence of regional variations of speech. Another drawback of Cued Speech is that the number of available Cued Speech transliterators (i.e., proficient cuers) is insufficient for the demand. In addition, children raised using Cued Speech without knowing ASL may not be able to communicate with the larger Deaf community of sign language users or those who use a form of English signing.

Some people also experience difficulties cueing at the normal pace of speech. Cued Speech does not guarantee an immediately adequate means of expression. In the United States, Cued Speech has received resistance from people supporting the communication philosophies of Bi-Bi or **Total Communication**. As suggested by Stewart and Lee (1987), "[I]t is unfortunate that Cornett chose to call Cued Speech a method of communication. This choice of terminology may have inadvertently put Cued Speech in competition with the full language based forms of other communication methods. In other words, it was placed in an all-or-none dilemma that educators and administrators felt compelled to resolve." (p. 61).

Generally speaking, Cued Speech is an efficient way of representing phonological information of a spoken language and provides a means of communicating this information to students who are deaf or hard of hearing. Through different handshapes and hand placements, Cued Speech produces a visual code representing the building blocks of a spoken language, thereby becoming a visual counterpart of speech. Despite its drawbacks, it has significant impact on the speech processing, oral language development, and literacy development of students who are deaf or hard of hearing.

Visual Phonics

Visual Phonics is the abbreviated title for See The Sound/Visual Phonics (STS/VP), which is a multisensory system consisting of 46 hand cues and corresponding written symbols that represents aspects of the phonemes of a language and the grapheme–phoneme relationships (phonics). This system was developed in 1982 by a mother of three deaf children and is distributed by the International Communication Learning Institute (ICLI) to help individuals with profound hearing loss gain access to phonological information of English. Visual Phonics was originally designed as a reading instructional tool for teaching letter–sound correspondences with the assumption that Visual Phonics use would fade when the students began to internalize the relationships. Currently, it is being used as an instructional tool to facilitate reading through the development of decoding skills, writing through the development of spelling and word study skills, and speech through the development of speech perception and articulation. Visual Phonics is neither a language nor a communication system; it is an instructional tool.

The hand cues of the Visual Phonics system are used in conjunction with spoken language and represent individual phonemes (sounds). Similar to Cued Speech, the speaker needs to maintain his or her hand near the mouth while speaking and cuing Visual Phonics simultaneously. The hand cues mirror the articulatory features of the sound, and the written symbols reflects the gestures used in the cues. For example, the cue for the voiced /th/ sound, as in the word *mother*, is produced by rubbing the index finger against the thumb with the other three fingers extended, representing the vibration of the tongue against the lips when producing this sound. On the other hand, the unvoiced /th/ sound, as in the word *teeth*, is produced using the same handshape, but the index finger is quickly lifted off the thumb representing the opening movement of the mouth that occurs when this sound is produced. The cue for the long vowel /o/, as in the word *bone*, is produced by making an *o* with the fingers and thumb like the *o* handshape in finger spelling and moving the hand outward from the mouth. The cue for the short vowel /o/, as in the word *top*, is very similar to the cue for the long vowel /o/, except it is produced using a flat *o* instead of a round *o*. Correspondingly, the written symbol for long vowel /o/ is a round *o*, and the one for short vowel /o/ is a flat *o*. These hand cues and written symbols offer a concrete way for children who are deaf

or hard of hearing to conceptualize the production of a sound and to link the sound to its printed correspondence.

The articulatory information in the hand cues is one of the major differences between Visual Phonics and Cued Speech. Essentially, Visual Phonics is used to prompt the articulatory feedback that will allow students to make use of the tactile-kinesthetic feedback system previously described. Once students learn the important articulatory features of the phonemes taught through the Visual Phonics hand cues, the cues tend to fade and students rely solely on articulatory feedback and thus the tactile-kinesthetic feedback system. As discussed previously, there is no articulatory information in the hand cues of Cued Speech. For example, in Cued Speech, the voiced /th/ as in *mother* is represented by Handshape 2 (index finger and middle finger) whereas the unvoiced /th/ sound as in *teeth* is represented by Handshape 7 (thumb, index finger, and middle finger). In other words, the handshapes utilized in Cued Speech contain no information to determine how the sound is produced.

Another distinctive feature of Visual Phonics is the written symbols that represent the handshapes. These written symbols provide visual discrimination between the letter and the sound it makes, which helps the student understand that the same letter or letter combination might make different sounds. When the student sees or writes the Visual Phonics symbols under the print words, he or she begins to identify patterns for letter–sound correspondence. The Visual Phonics written symbols have obvious advantages over the **International Phonetic Alphabet (IPA)** because the Visual Phonics symbols are based on the production of the hand cues and are dramatically different from the print letters whereas many IPA symbols are identical to the English letters.

Visual Phonics provides children who are deaf or hard of hearing with mental images of phonemes, and such a phonological representation of English directly assists the students in manipulating the phonemes and acquiring phonemic awareness and phonics skills. This multimodal representation of phonemes can be used to assist students who are deaf or hard of hearing or other struggling readers who experience difficulties to appropriately and adequately access the phonological components of English language. Visual Phonics can be used with any communication methodology because it is an instructional tool instead of a communication system.

Even though Visual Phonics has been implemented in the field for 25 years, only a few empirical research studies have been conducted to evaluate its efficiency in assisting the phonological development of students who are deaf or hard of hearing. Trezek and her colleagues (Trezek & Malmgren, 2005; Trezek & Wang, 2006; Trezek, Wang, Woods, Gampp, & Paul, 2007) conducted a series of pioneer studies and reported the effectiveness of various phonics treatment packages incorporating Visual Phonics in teaching phonological processing skills to early elementary students and middle school students who are deaf or hard of hearing. These studies as well as others are explored in greater detail in Chapter 4.

A summary of a pilot study evaluating the effectiveness of Visual Phonics integrated into reading instruction for hearing kindergarten students is available as part of the training materials distributed by ICLI (Slauson & Carrier, 1996). In this study, kindergarten students in the treatment group received phonics instruction supplemented by Visual Phonics. After six months of instruction, treatment students showed significantly greater gains on measures of letter recognition, sound association, and reading words when compared to control students who were not exposed to Visual Phonics.

In addition to this summary, training materials also include information regarding studies evaluating the effectiveness of Visual Phonics as it relates to improvements in speech intelligibility in children with Down syndrome (Smith-Stubblefield & Guidi, 1996) and individuals with developmental apraxia (Engel & Murray, 1996. Wilson-Favors (1987) also conducted a preliminarily study with six 10- to 12-year-old deaf students with unintelligible speech. At the beginning of the school year, all six participants were given the Fisher Logemann Test of Articulation Competence (Fisher & Logemann, 1971), and the sounds that were frequently misarticulated or left out were selected as targets for instruction. Each student set a goal of three to six sounds. After one year of group speech sessions using Visual Phonics, all six students showed progress in the correct articulation of their target sounds without cues, and they were all able to articulate more target sounds when hand cues were given.

Visual Phonics is a promising instructional tool to assist students in reading, writing, and speech development. Not only students who are deaf or hard of hearing, but also other struggling readers can obtain potential benefits from this alternative access to phonological information. Despite its potential promise, Visual Phonics has some of the same weaknesses that were discussed relative to Cued Speech such as the problem of interindividual and intraindividual consistency, which might be a universal issue in any cuing system. Long-term intervention research is needed in the field to further assess the effectiveness of Visual Phonics as an instructional tool. In addition, more research is needed from the perspective of teacher training for implementing Visual Phonics in the classroom. We cannot emphasize enough that Visual Phonics alone cannot provide sufficient support for students' phonological development. Visual Phonics needs to be grounded in a systematic and explicit phonics program such as the Direct Instruction *Corrective Reading-Decoding* (Trezek & Malmgren, 2005) or *Reading Mastery* (Trezek & Wang, 2006) series to yield the maximum positive results. Once again, Visual Phonics is only a supplementary instructional tool, not an entire reading curriculum.

In sum, four major alternative means of acquiring phonology have been discussed: speech reading, articulatory feedback, Cued Speech, and Visual Phonics. Speech reading is generally considered to be insufficient in capturing phonological information in a spoken language; however, articulatory feedback, Cued Speech, and Visual Phonics provide some promising evidence of assisting students who are deaf or hard of hearing in acquiring phonological information from a spoken language.

CONCLUSION

The purpose of this chapter was to discuss research on phonology and deafness. We started with the definition of working memory and the role of working memory in the reading process. Next, we discussed the definition of phonology and its related terms, as well as the role of phonological processing in reading. We provided a brief review of literature on phonological coding of deaf readers and concluded that, despite some counterevidence, the general agreement in the field is that deaf readers, particularly skilled deaf readers, have access to phonological information. This conclusion confirms the previous pattern we identified regarding reading development in general: Students who are deaf or hard of hearing are qualitatively similar and quantitatively delayed in phonological awareness development. To

address the limited access to phonology for students who are deaf or hard of hearing, several alternative means for acquiring phonology are available. We discussed four major methods in detail: speech reading, articulatory feedback, Cued Speech, and Visual Phonics.

CHAPTER SUMMARY

- Working memory is a limited-capacity mental system responsible for the temporary storage and processing of information necessary to handle tasks that require comprehension, learning, and reasoning. During the reading process, working memory is responsible for simultaneously retaining information just read as well as processing previously read information.

- Orthographic, phonological, semantic, and contextual analysis of the print word should occur simultaneously during reading, and students need to be directly taught to conduct these analyses in concert with one another.

- Although still controversial, substantial research has suggested that deaf readers, particularly skilled readers, have access to phonological information. Compared to their hearing peers, students who are deaf or hard of hearing are qualitatively similar yet quantitatively delayed in their phonological awareness development.

- Alternative means of acquiring phonology for students who are deaf or hard of hearing include speech reading, articulatory feedback, Cued Speech, and Visual Phonics.

- Phonological processing is able to enhance the capacity of working memory, and working memory plays a critical role for storing and processing information during reading.

REVIEW QUESTIONS

1. What is working memory? What is the role of working memory in reading?

2. What are the five types of internal coding strategies that are used by deaf individuals in working memory?

3. Briefly describe the following terms:

    (a) Phonology

    (b) Phonemes

    (c) Knowledge of the alphabetic principle

4. What is the role of phonology in reading?

5. What are the general findings on phonological coding for deaf readers?

6. What are the four alternative means of acquiring phonology for students who are deaf or hard of hearing as discussed in this chapter? Briefly describe each method.

REFLECTIVE QUESTIONS

1. According to Bilingual/Bicultural (Bi-Bi) programs supported by the notion of a Deaf epistemology, it is possible to proceed from ASL to the written form of English directly—that is, individuals with skills acquired in ASL can bypass the performance form (i.e., spoken and/or signed) of English and still acquire the ability to read and write in English. Do you agree with this assumption? Why or why not?

2. Manually coded English systems (e.g., signed English, signing exact English) were designed to visually represent the structure of English. What are the advantages or disadvantages (or both) of utilizing these manually coded English systems in reading instruction for students who are deaf or hard of hearing?

3. Comparing Cued Speech and Visual Phonics as reading instructional tools for students who are deaf or hard of hearing, what are their advantages and disadvantages?

SUGGESTED READINGS AND RESOURCES

Bradley, L., & Bryant, P. (1985). *Rhyme and reason in reading and spelling*. Ann Arbor: University of Michigan Press.

Deland, F. (1968). *The story of lip-reading*. Washington, DC: Volta Bureau.

Goldstein, M. (1939). *The acoustic method*. St. Louis: Laryngoscope Press.

O'Rourke, T. J. (1972). *Psycholinguistics and total communication: The state of the art*. Silver Spring, MD: American Annals of the Deaf.

Weiner, F. (1979). *Phonological process analysis*. Baltimore: University Park Press.

REFERENCES

Adams, M. (1990). *Beginning to read: Thinking and learning about print.* Cambridge: MIT Press.

Adams, M. (2004). Modeling the connections between word recognition and reading. In R. B. Ruddell & N. Unrau (Eds.), *Theoretical models and processes of reading* (5th. ed.) (pp. 1219–1243). Newark, DE: International Reading Association.

Alegria, J. (1998). The origin and functions of phonological representations in deaf people. In C. Hulme & R. M. Joshi (Eds.), *Reading and spelling: Development and disorders* (pp. 263–286). Mahwah, NJ: Erlbaum.

Alegria, J., Charlier, B., & Mattys, S. (1999). The role of lipreading and Cued-Speech in the processing of phonological information in French-educated deaf children. *European Journal of Cognitive Psychology, 11,* 451–472.

Alegria, J., & Lechat, J. (2005). Phonological processing in deaf children: When lipreading and cues are incongruent. *Journal of Deaf Studies and Deaf Education, 10* (2), 122–133.

Baddeley, A. (1986). *Working memory.* Oxford: Clarendon Press.

Baddeley, A. (1990). *Human memory: Theory and practice.* Hillsdale, NJ: Lawrence Erlbaum.

Boutla, M., Supalla, T. Newport, E. L., & Bavelier, D. (2004). Short-term memory span: Insights from sign language. *Nature Neuroscience, 7* (9), 997–1002.

Chall, J. S. (1996). *Stages of reading development.* (2nd ed.). New York: McGraw-Hill.

Charlier, B. L., & Leybaert, J. (2000). The rhyming skills of deaf children educated with phonetically augmented speechreading. *Quarterly Journal of Experimental Psychology, 53A,* 349–375.

Cheng, A. K., Grant, G. D., & Niparko, J. K. (1999). Meta-analysis of pediatric cochlear implant literature. *Annals of Otology, Rhinology & Laryngology: Supplement, 177,* 124–128.

Clarke, R. B., & Ling, D. (1976). The effects of using Cued Speech: A follow-up study. *The Volta Review, 78,* 123–134.

Colin, S., Magnan, A., Ecalle, J., & Leybaert, J. (2007). Relation between deaf children's phonological skills in kindergarten and word recognition performance in first grade. *Journal of Child Psychology and Psychiatry, 48* (2), 139–146.

Connor, C. M., & Zwolan, T. A. (2004). Examining multiple sources of influence on the reading comprehension skills of children who use cochlear implants. *Journal of Speech, Language, and Hearing Research, 47* (3), 509–526.

Conrad, R. (1979). *The deaf schoolchild: Language and cognitive function.* London: Harper & Row.

Cornett, R. O. (1967). Cued Speech. *American Annals of the Deaf, 112,* 3–13.

Cornett, R. O., & Daisey, M. (1992). *The Cued Speech resource book for parents of deaf children.* Raleigh, NC: National Cued Speech Corporation.

Cummins, J. (1989). A theoretical framework for bilingual special education. *Exceptional Children, 56,* 111–119.

Dyer, A., MacSweeney, M., Szczerbinski, M., Green. L., & Campbell, R. (2003). Predictor of reading delay in deaf adolescences: The relative contribution of Rapid Automatized Naming speed and phonological awareness and decoding. *Journal of Deaf Studies and Deaf Education*, 8 (3), 215–229.

Engel, D. C. & Murray, K. (1996). *An application of Visual Phonics in treatment of Development Apraxia*. Training materials from International Communication Learning Institute, Webster, WI. See the Sound Visual Phonics Research and Articles.

Ewoldt, C. (1996). Deaf bilingualism: A holistic perspective. *Australian Journal of the Education of the Deaf*, 2, 5–9.

Fagan, M., Pisoni, D., Horn, D., & Dillion, C. (2007). Neuropsychological correlates of vocabulary, reading, and working memory in deaf children with cochlear implants. *Journal of Deaf Studies and Deaf Education*, 12 (4), 461–471.

Fisher, H., & Logemann, J. (1971). *Fisher Logemann Test of Articulation Competence*. Australia: Pro-ed.

Fleetwood, E., & Metzger, M. (1998). *Cued language structure: An analysis of cued American English based on linguistic principles*. Silver Spring, MD: Calliope Press.

Gallaudet Research Institute (2005, December). *Regional and National Summary Report of Data from the 2004–2005 Annual Survey of Deaf and Hard of Hearing Children and Youth*. Washington, DC: GRI, Gallaudet University.

Gathercole, S., & Baddeley, A. (1989). Development of vocabulary in children and short-term phonological memory. *Journal of Memory and Language*, 28, 200–213.

Gathercole, S., & Baddeley, A. (1990). Phonological memory deficits in language disordered children: Is there a causal connection? *Journal of Memory and Language, 29*, 336–360.

Geers, A. E. (2002). Factors affecting the development of speech, language, and literacy in children with cochlear implants. *Language, Speech, and Hearing Services in Schools, 33*, 172–183.

Geers, A. E. (2003). Predictors of reading skill development in children with early cochlear implantations. *Ear & Hearing, 24* (1S), 59S–68S.

Geers, A. E. (2004). Speech, language, and reading skills after early cochlear implantation. *Archives of Otolaryngology—Head and Neck Surgery, 130* (5), 634–638.

Geers, A. E., Nicholas, J., & Sedey, A. L. (2003). Language skills of children with early cochlear implantation. *Ear & Hearing, 24* (1S), 46S–58S.

Hanson, V. L. (1991). Phonological processing without sound. In S. A. Brady & D. P. Shankweiler (Eds.), *Phonological processes in literacy: A tribute to Isabelle Y. Liberman* (pp. 153–162). Hillsdale, NJ: Erlbaum.

Hanson, V. L., Goodell, E. W., & Perfetti, C. A. (1991). Tongue-twister effects in the silent reading of hearing and deaf college students. *Journal of Memory and Language, 30*, 319–330.

Hanson, V. L., Liberman, I. Y., & Shankweiler, D. (1984). Linguistic coding by deaf children in relation to beginning reading success. *Journal of Experimental Child Psychology, 37*, 378–393.

Hanson, V. L., & Wilkenfeld, D. (1985). Morphophonology and lexical organization in deaf readers. *Language and Speech, 18*, 269–280.

Houston, D. M., Carter, A. K., Pisoni, D. B., Kirk, K. I., & Ying, E. A. (2005). Word learning in children following cochlear implantation. *The Volta Review, 105* (1), 41–72.

Izzo, A. (2002). Phonemic awareness and reading ability: An investigation with young readers who are deaf. *American Annals of the Deaf, 147* (4), 18–28.

Johnson, H. A., Padak, N. D., & Barton, L. E. (1994). Developmental spelling strategies of hearing-impaired children. *Reading and Writing Quarterly, 10,* 359–367.

Kelly, L. (1993). Recall of English function words and inflections by skilled and average deaf readers. *American Annals of the Deaf, 138,* 288–296.

Kyllo, K. L. (2003). Phonemic awareness through immersion in cued American English. *Odyssey, 5* (1), 36–44.

LaSasso, C. (1996). Fonicks for deff tshildrun? Yoo beddzah! *Perspectives in Education and Deafness, 14,* 6–9.

LaSasso, C., & Crain, K. L. (2003). Research and theory support Cued Speech. *Odyssey, 5* (1), 30–35.

LaSasso, C., Crain, K. L., & Leybaert, J. (2003). Rhyme generation in deaf students: The effect of exposure to Cued Speech. *Journal of Deaf Studies and Deaf Education, 8* (3), 250–270.

LaSasso, C. J., & Metzger, M. A. (1998). An alternate route for preparing deaf children for BiBi programs: The home language as L1 and Cued Speech for conveying traditionally spoken languages. *Journal of Deaf Studies and Deaf Education, 3* (4), 265–289.

Leybaert, J. (1993). Reading in the deaf: The roles of phonological codes. In M. Marschark & M. D. Clark (Eds.), *Psychological Perspectives on Deafness* (pp. 269–309). Hillsdale, NJ: Lawrence Erlbaum Associates.

Leybaert, J. (1998). Phonological representations in deaf children: the importance of early linguistic experience. *Scandinavian Journal of Psychology, 39,* 169–173.

Leybaert, J. (2000). Phonology acquired through the eyes and spelling in deaf children. *Journal of Experimental Child Psychology, 75,* 291–318.

Leybaert, J., Alegria, J., Hage, C., & Charlier, B. (1998). The effect of exposure to phonetically augmented lip speech in the prelingual deaf. In R. Campbell, B. Dodd, and D. Burham (Eds.), *Hearing by eye II: Advances in the psychology of speech-reading and auditory-visual speech* (pp. 283–301). Hove, England: Psychology Press.

Leybaert, J., & Charlier, B. (1996). Visual speech in the head: the effect of Cued-Speech on rhyming, remembering, and spelling. *Journal of Deaf Studies and Deaf Education, 1* (4), 234–248.

Leybaert, J., & Lechat, J. (2001a). Phonological similarity effects in memory for serial order of Cued Speech. *Journal of Speech, Language and Hearing Research, 44,* 949–963.

Leybaert, J., & Lechat, J. (2001b). Variability in deaf children's spelling: The effect of language experience. *Journal of Educational Psychology, 93* (3), 554–562.

Ling, D., & Clarke, B. R. (1975). Cued Speech: An evaluative study. *American Annals of the Deaf, 120* (5), 480–488.

Livingston, S. (1997). *Rethinking the education of deaf students.* Portsmouth, NH: Heinemann.

Luetke-Stahlman, B., & Nielsen, D. C. (2003). The contribution of phonological awareness and receptive and expressive English to the reading ability of deaf students with varying degree of exposure to accurate

English. *Journal of Deaf Studies and Deaf Education, 8* (4), 464–484.

Marschark, M., & Harris, M. (1996). Success and failure in learning to read: The special case (?) of deaf children. In C. Cornoldi & J. Oakhill (Eds.), *Reading comprehension difficulties: Processes and intervention* (pp. 279–300). Mahwah, NJ: Erlbaum.

Marschark, M., Rhoten, C., & Fabich, M. (2007). Effects of cochlear implants on children's reading and academic achievement. *Journal of Deaf Studies and Deaf Education, 12* (3), 269–282.

McGurk, H., & MacDonald, J. (1976). Hearing lips and seeing voices. *Nature, 264,* 746–748.

Miller, G. A. (1956). The magic number seven, plus or minus two: Some limits on our capacity for processing information. *Psychology Review, 63,* 81–97.

Miller, P. (2002). Communication mode and the processing of printed words: Evidence from readers with prelingually acquired deafness. *Journal of Deaf Studies and Deaf Education, 7* (4), 312–329.

Miller, P. (2004). Processing of written word and nonword visual information by individuals with prelingual deafness. *Journal of Speech, Language, and Hearing Research, 47,* 990–1000.

Miyamoto, R. T., Svirsky, M. A., & Robbins, A. (1997). Enhancement of expressive language in prelingually deaf children with cochlear implants. *Acta Oto-Laryngologica, 117,* 154–157.

Moog, J. S. (2002). Changing expectations for children with cochlear implants. *Annals of Otology, Rhinology, and Laryngology—Supplement, 189,* 138–142.

Moores, D. F. (1969). Cued Speech: Some practical and theoretical considerations. *American Annals of the Deaf, 114,* 1, 23–33.

Moores, D. F. (2006). Print literacy: The acquisition of reading and writing skills, in D. F. Moores & D. S. Martin (Eds.) *Deaf Learners* (pp. 41–55), Washington, DC: Gallaudet University Press.

National Cued Speech Association. (2007, October 13). *Special Populations.* Retrieved October 13, 2007, from http://www.cuedspeech.org/sub/cued/uses.asp

National Reading Panel (2000). *Report of the National Reading Panel: Teaching children to read—An evidence-based Assessment of the scientific research literature on reading and its implications for reading instruction.* Jessup, MD: National Institute for Literacy at EDPubs.

Nicholls, G. H., & Ling, D. (1982). Cued speech and the reception of spoken language. *Journal of Speech and Hearing Research, 25,* 262–269.

Paul, P. (1990). Using ASL to teach English literacy skills. *The Deaf American, 40* (1–4), 107–113.

Paul, P. (2001). *Language and deafness* (3rd ed.). San Diego: Singular Publishing Group.

Paul, P., Bernhardt, E., & Gramley, C. (1992). Use of ASL in teaching reading and writing to deaf students: An interactive theoretical perspective. In *Conference Proceedings: Bilingual Considerations in the Education of Deaf Students: ASL and English* (pp. 75–105). Washington, DC: Gallaudet University, Extension and Summer Programs.

Perfetti, C. A., & Sandak, R. (2000). Reading optimally builds on spoken language: Implications for deaf readers. *Journal of Deaf Studies and Deaf Education, 5* (1), 32–50.

Reagan, T. (1985). The deaf as a linguistic minority: Educational considerations. *Harvard Educational Review, 55,* 265–277.

Schirmer, B. R., & McGough, S. M. (2005). Teaching reading to children who are deaf: Do the conclusions of the National Reading Panel apply? *Review of Educational Research, 75* (1), 83–117.

Schirmer, B. R., & Williams, C. (2003). Approaches to teaching reading. In M. Marschark & P. Spencer (Eds.), *Handbook of deaf studies, language, and education* (110–122). New York: Oxford University Press.

Slauson, V. & Carrier, J. (1996). *Making phonics multisensory: Using the See the Sound/Visual Phonics to enhance early reading instruction.* Training materials from International Communication Learning Institute, Webster, WI. See the Sound Visual Phonics Research and Articles.

Smith-Stubblefield, S. & Guidi, K. (1996). *A facilitating technique to improve speech intelligibility in individuals with Down's Syndrome.* Retrieved October 17, 2007, from http://www.altonweb.com/cs/down-syndrome/index.htm?page=visualphonics.html

Snow, C., Burns, S., & Griffin, P. (Eds.). (1998). *Preventing reading difficulties in young children.* Washington, DC: National Academy Press.

Snowling, M., & Hulme, C. (Eds.). (2005). *The science of reading: A handbook.* Malden, MA: Blackwell.

Spencer, L., Barker, B. A., & Tomblin, J. B. (2003). Exploring the language and literacy outcomes of pediatric cochlear implant users. *Ear & Hearing, 24* (3), 236–247.

Spencer, L., Tomblin, J. B., & Gantz, B. J. (1997). Reading skills in children with multichannel cochlear implant experience. *The Volta Review, 99* (4), 193–202.

Stewart, D. A., & Lee, B. B. (1987). Cued Speech revisited. *B.C. Journal of Special Education, 11* (1), 57–63.

Strong, M. (1988). A bilingual approach to the education of young deaf children: ASL and English. In M. Strong (Ed.), *Language learning and deafness* (pp. 113–129). New York: Cambridge University Press.

Sutcliffe, A., Dowker, A., & Campbell, R. (1999). Deaf children's spelling: Does it show sensitivity to phonology? *Journal of Deaf Studies and Deaf Education, 4* (2), 111–123.

Tierney, R. (1994). Dissension, tensions, the models of literacy. In R. Ruddell, M. Ruddell, & H. Singer (Eds.), *Theoretical models and processes of reading* (4th ed.) (pp. 1162–1182). Newark, DE: International Reading Association.

Tomblin, J. B., Spencer, L., Flock, S., Tyler, R., & Gantz, B. (1999). A comparison of language achievement in children with cochlear implants and children using hearing aids, *Journal of Speech, Language, and Hearing Research, 42* (2), 497–511.

Trezek, B. J., & Malmgren, K. W. (2005). The efficacy of utilizing a phonics treatment package with middle school deaf and hard-of-hearing students. *Journal of Deaf Studies and Deaf Education, 10* (3), 256–271.

Trezek, B. J. & Wang, Y. (2006). Implications of utilizing a phonics-based reading curriculum with children who are deaf or hard of hearing. *Journal of Deaf Studies and Deaf Education, 11* (2), 202–213.

Trezek, B. J., Wang, Y., Woods, D. G., Gampp, T. L., & Paul, P. (2007). Using Visual Phonics to supplement beginning reading instruction for students who are deaf or hard of hearing. *Journal of Deaf*

Studies and Deaf Education, 12 (3), 373–384.

Tye-Murray, N., Spencer, L., & Woodworth, G. (1995). Acquisition of speech by children who have prolonged cochlear implant experience. *Journal of Speech and Hearing Research, 38,* 327–337.

Vermeulen, A., van Bon, W., Schreuder, R., Knoors, H., & Snik, A. (2007). Reading comprehension of deaf children with cochlear implants. *Journal of Deaf Studies and Deaf Education. 12* (3), 283–302.

Vieu, A., Mondain, M., Blanchard, K., Sillon, M., Reuillard-Artieres, F., Tobey, E., Uziel, A., & Piron, J. P. (1998). Influence of communication mode on speech intelligibility and syntactic structure of sentences in profoundly hearing impaired French children implanted between 5 and 9 years of age. *International*

Journal of Pediatric Otorhinolaryngology, 44, 15–22.

Vygotsky, L. (1962). *Thought and language.* Cambridge: MIT Press.

Vygotsky, L. (1978). *Mind in society: The development of higher psychological processes.* Cambridge, MA: Harvard University Press.

Willstedt-Svensson, U., Lofqvist, A., Almqvist, B., & Sahlen, B. (2004). Is age at implant the only factor that counts? The influence of working memory on lexical and grammatical development in children with cochlear implants. *International Journal of Audiology, 43,* 506–515.

Wilson-Favors, V. (1987, November/December). Using the visual phonics system to improve speech skills: A preliminary study. *Perspectives in Education and Deafness, 6* (2), 2–4.

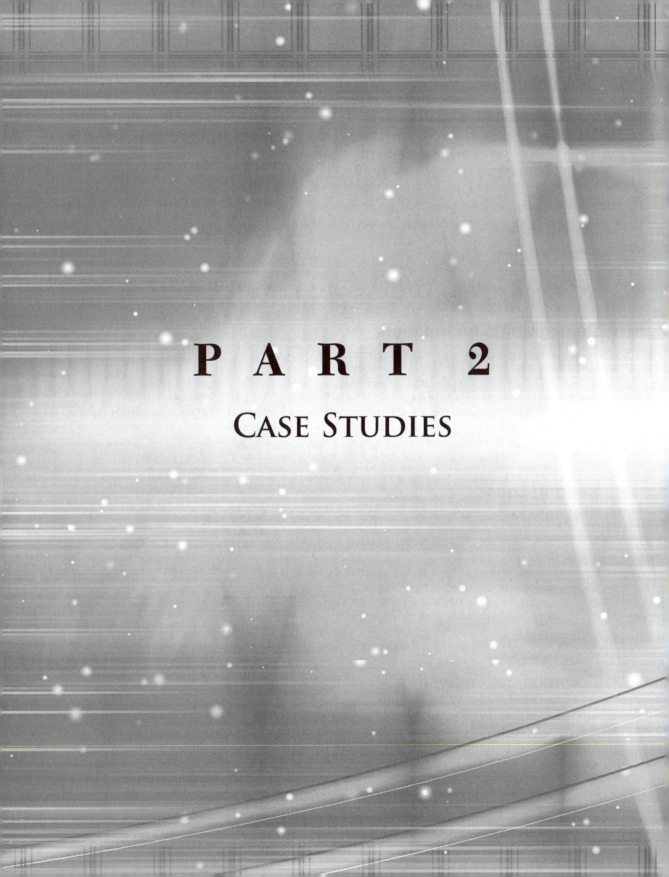

PART 2
CASE STUDIES

CASE STUDIES

In this section of the book, we introduce you to four students who are deaf or hard of hearing. For each student, we provide you with the following: (1) demographic information, (2) degree of hearing loss, (3) type of communication system, (4) academic history and present level of performance in reading, and (5) other relevant information. In Chapters 4 through 7 of this text, we will offer you the opportunity to apply knowledge and skills gained in these chapters to address the reading instructional needs of the four students. In subsequent chapters, we will refer you to the Case Studies included here and ask that you complete several Application Exercises related to these students.

CASE STUDY A: AIDAN

Demographic Information

Aidan is a 6-year-old student who attends kindergarten in a regional program for students who are deaf or hard of hearing in a suburban public school district. Aidan is the youngest of two children; he and his 9-year-old hearing sister, Madison, reside with their parents, Julie and Mike, on the west side of town. Julie is a part-time real estate agent, whereas Mike is employed as an accountant for the local telecommunications company. Although Aidan and Madison both attend school in their local school district, Madison is enrolled in the neighborhood school on the west side but Aidan attends school on the east side of town. Daily transportation to and from the school, where the regional program is located, is provided by the school district. Because Julie is currently employed part-time, she is at home when the children return from school each day.

Hearing Loss

Aidan's hearing loss was first suspected when he failed his newborn hearing screening. There is no family history of hearing loss. Follow-up appointments with an audiologist during his infancy confirmed a severe, bilateral, sensorineural hearing loss 70/75/80 dB HL at 500, 1000, and 2000 Hz. Although Aidan began wearing hearing aids at 9 months of age, consistent use did not begin until age 2. Even though his aided thresholds appear to provide him with access to the majority of speech sounds, Aidan's speech production is characterized by many omissions and substitutions, particularly in the high-frequency range. Aidan's speech is thus unintelligible to unfamiliar listeners, although familiar listeners such as family members and teachers report that his speech is typically understood when using common phrases or when the context of his message is known. Aidan has received hearing evaluations at least annually since his loss was identified, and his hearing aids have been maintained on a consistent schedule.

Communication System

The regional program for students who are deaf or hard of hearing where Aidan attends school has adopted a total communication philosophy. Simultaneous communication and Conceptually Accurate Signed English (CASE) is employed by teachers during instructional activities. Teachers describe CASE as using conceptually accurate signs derived from American Sign Language in an English sentence order (i.e., English syntax). For example, in CASE one sign is used to indicate the two English words "stand up" rather than two separate signs. The teachers also explained that articles (*a, an, the*) and endings (*-ed, -ing*) are incorporated into instructional activities using finger spelling, but they are not typically utilized during conversation. Sound field amplification systems are installed in the classrooms at Aidan's school.

Aidan's parents began attending sign language classes offered by the school district once a week when Aidan was 18 months old. Although Julie and Mike attended regularly until Aidan was 3-years-old, their attendance over the past three years has been inconsistent. At home, Aidan and his family rely primarily on speech and basic signs for communication. His parents state that when Aidan is confused or does not understand their message aurally, they often provide a few signs or finger spell key words. His parents admit that they are basic signers and will probably need to improve their skills as Aidan ages in order to assist him with his homework. Aidan and Madison, along with their parents, occasionally attend family events offered by the local deaf club.

Academic History and Present Level of Performance

Aidan began receiving services through early intervention at the age of nine months and received early childhood services in a classroom setting beginning at age 3. In kindergarten, Aidan spends the majority of his school day in a self-contained classroom taught by a teacher of the deaf and hard of hearing. He and his classmates are included in the general education environment with the assistance of both a teacher of the deaf and hard of hearing and an interpreter for activities and subjects that are deemed appropriate for the students. During instructional classes such as physical education and Art, Aidan and his classmates attend sessions with their hearing peers and are provided with an interpreter. Aidan also receives services from the school's speech and language clinician three times a week for 15-minute sessions.

Ongoing assessments of Aidan's speech and language skills indicate that his skills are delayed when compared to the developmental milestones for students who are hearing. In particular, his spontaneous spoken and signed language is fairly simplistic and ranges from three- to five-word utterances. In addition, he rarely uses adjectives or adverbs when describing objects or actions, but he will do so when prompted by an adult. Through modeling, his teachers are beginning to require him to both sign and verbalize complete English sentences as a means of increasing his mean length of utterance. Aidan has a good grasp of basic temporal concepts such as *today*, *tomorrow*, and *yesterday*, but he continues to struggle with the concept of *week* and *month* despite extensive instruction. Aidan is able to name and describe the use for many common objects and is beginning to include articles when referring to them.

Aidan's teachers recently received training in Visual Phonics and began to incorporate this supplement into reading instructional activities last year. The teachers sought the training because the school's mandated basal reading series contains a strong phonemic component and, without Visual Phonics, they were uncertain how to utilize the curriculum with students. Aidan's teachers recently administered the Letter-Word Identification, Word Attack, Reading Comprehension and Spelling of Sounds subtests of the Woodcock Johnson Test of Achievement-III to all kindergarten students enrolled in the regional program. This assessment will be administered again at the end of the school year to indicate students' progress.

Results of this assessment indicate that although Aidan knows many letter–sound correspondences, he has difficulty blending and segmenting sounds and therefore applying this knowledge to reading and spelling activities. When successful blending does occur, Aidan can often verbally produce the resulting word and the correct Visual Phonics cues, but he is not able to indicate the meaning of the word by providing a sign or description. His teachers indicate that Aidan requires much more repetition than his peers to acquire new vocabulary; therefore, his parents are often asked to practice the new vocabulary with him at home. His sister, Madison, enjoys assisting Aidan with these vocabulary activities, and she is working with him to create a personal, pictorial dictionary for the words his teachers send home.

Other

Aidan has been involved in the local park district's soccer program for the past year. He enjoys the practice sessions but not participating in the games. His mother reports that the structured practice sessions allow Aidan to participate fairly readily, but his hearing loss makes it difficult for him to follow his coach's and fellow teammates' directives while on the field. Aidan's mother has been discussing this situation with the administrators of the park district and has requested that an interpreter be provided for Aidan.

CASE STUDY B: BRIANNA

Demographic Information

Brianna is a 9-year-old fourth grade student living with her family in a community with a population of approximately 40,000 located 65 miles from a large, urban area. Brianna has two older siblings: a brother, Matthew, who is a freshman in high school, and a sister, Caroline, who is in seventh grade. There is no history of hearing loss on either side of her family. Brianna's parents, Jeff and Michelle, have been divorced for three years. Michelle has primary custody of the three children during the school year. The children live with her during the week and visit their father every other weekend. Jeff and Michelle share custody of the children during the summer months. The community where the family lives is home to a state university, where both of Brianna's parents are employed. Jeff is an associate professor in the business school, and Michelle is employed in graduate admissions.

Hearing Loss

Brianna's severe to profound, bilateral sensorineural hearing loss was identified when she was 9 months of age, and she began using amplification immediately. When Brianna was 18-months-old, her parents began investigating a cochlear implant, and she underwent the surgical procedure at the age of 2½ years. Brianna's surgery was conducted at the children's hospital in the city 65 miles from their home, and follow-up mapping appointments were performed there for the first year. However, Brianna's therapy has always been performed locally at the audiology and speech clinic housed at the university where her parents are employed. According to her therapists and parents, Brianna has made wonderful progress with her implant.

Communication System

Brianna utilizes oral and aural skills to communicate in all situations and does not know sign language.

Academic History and Present Level of Performance

Brianna began attending preschool in her local school district at age 3. Since beginning kindergarten, she has attended her neighborhood school and received itinerant services from a teacher of the deaf and hard of hearing through the local special education cooperative. Brianna's service has varied over the years, but she is currently receiving 30 minutes of service three times a week from the itinerant teacher of the deaf and hard of hearing and 30 minutes of service two times a week from the school-based speech and language clinician. These professionals work collaboratively to achieve the goals outlined in Brianna's individual education program and meet regularly to discuss her progress.

Sessions with the itinerant teacher of the deaf and hard of hearing and the speech and language clinician focus primarily on supporting Brianna's placement in general education curriculum and instruction. At the beginning of each school year, the itinerant teacher conducts an inservice for Brianna's homeroom teacher to describe her cochlear implant and the accommodations and support that are needed. The speech and language clinician serves as Brianna's case manager because she is present at the school on a daily basis.

In the area of reading, Brianna has strong decoding skills and is a good speller, but she struggles with acquiring new vocabulary and comprehension tasks that require abstract thought. Assessments conducted in the fall of her fourth-grade year also indicate that her reading fluency was below the 25th percentile when compared to national norms. Although she can decode the majority of words in grade-level passages, she experiences difficulty with phrasing and expression. Brianna's labored reading may also contribute to the difficulties she has with reading comprehension because she reports that she often has trouble remembering what she has read.

In addition to reading fluency exercises, Brianna benefits from direct vocabulary instruction, particularly content-specific vocabulary and instruction in base words and affixes. She also requires instruction in using various comprehension strategies and benefits from the use of graphic organizers that allow her to manage abstract ideas in a hand-on, concrete manner. Brianna's fourth-grade teacher reports that she provides her with preferential seating and that she appears to perform best when visual aids are used to support instruction. Her teacher states that she struggles with cooperative group activities, but the teacher is uncertain whether Brianna's hearing loss, knowledge of the content, or shy personality contributes to the difficulties she experiences.

Other

Despite her reported shyness, Brianna is an active member of her local Girl Scout troop and appears to have several close friends. Brianna took swimming lessons offered through the park district this past summer and is considering joining the competitive swim team next summer. Because she is unable to wear her implant when swimming, Brianna is concerned about how she will negotiate being a member of a team that requires her to communicate with her coach and teammates. She has asked that her itinerant teacher and speech and language clinician assist her in developing strategies for communicating in these situations.

CASE STUDY C: CARLOS

Demographic Information

Carlos is a 15-year-old high school freshman living in an urban area. The district in which he attends school has a total student population of 420,982. Demographics of the district are 48.6% African-American, 37.6% Latino, 8.1% Caucasian, 3.2% Asian or Pacific Islander, 2.4% multiracial, and 0.1% Native American. According to the annual report published by the district, 85.6% of students are from low-income families and 13.7% are limited-English-proficient.

Carlos' parents Juan and Maria are originally from Mexico. Soon after Carlos was born, his family relocated to the United States. His family originally lived in Texas before moving to the Midwest to be closer to Maria's sisters. Carlos is the youngest of four children, all of whom are boys. Two of the four boys have completed high school and no longer live in the family home. Carlos' brother Manuel is a senior in high school and still lives at home with Carlos and his parents. Juan is an assistant manager at a local produce store, and Maria is employed by a large hotel franchise downtown.

The neighborhood in which Carlos lives has a strong Latino influence. Many of the local businesses use advertisements written in Spanish, and the majority of business is conducted in Spanish as well. Although Juan and Maria know some English, Spanish is the primary language spoken in the home. Carlos' parents prefer to have a Spanish translator provided when attending school functions and meetings.

Hearing Loss

Carlos's hearing loss was identified at age 3 when he failed a hearing screening while attending Head Start preschool. There is no prior history of hearing loss in the family. Carlos's parents, however, report that he became very ill soon after they relocated to the United States. Carlos had a high fever that lasted for several days, and his parents suspect that this illness may have resulted in his hearing loss. An audiological exam at age 3 confirmed a moderate, bilateral, sensorineural hearing loss. The configuration of his hearing loss is unique with 0/40/80 dB HL at 500, 1000, and 2000 Hz for his right ear and 40/40/40 at 500, 1000, and 2000 Hz for his left ear. Given the configuration of the loss in the right ear, Carlos uses only one hearing aid in his left ear. Carlos also has a history of severe ear infections; therefore, a conductive hearing loss component is often present and sometimes reduces his ability to make good use of his residual hearing. When he was younger, Carlos had tubes in his ears. Although this seemed to reduce the prevalence of ear infections, he continues to have at least three episodes a year.

Communication System

Carlos uses oral language as his primary mode of communication. However, because he attends school at the same site where the district's hearing impaired program is housed, Carlos has been exposed to sign language since preschool. Although his expressive sign language skills are weak, he benefits greatly from using sign language receptively. This is particularly true in instances when he is experiencing an ear infection. Carlos uses Spanish to communicate at home and in his community.

Academic History and Present Level of Performance

As previously noted, Carlos's hearing loss was identified when he was attending preschool at Head Start. After his diagnosis at age 3, Carlos began receiving services through his local school district's hearing-impaired program. Carlos was involved in the district's self-contained program through kindergarten. Beginning in first grade, he was included in the general education environment for all subjects expect for reading and language. In the general education environment, Carlos had received support from a teacher of the deaf in a resource setting.

This educational arrangement has continued throughout the years. Now that he is in high school, Carlos attends general education classes in English, social studies, and science. The section of the English class in which he is enrolled is team taught. In this instance, the general education teacher works collaboratively with a special educator to provide instruction and accommodations. This year, Carlos and two other students who are deaf or hard of hearing are enrolled in this special section of English class and are provided with an educational interpreter.

As part of his seven-day class schedule, Carlos also receives additional support from a teacher of the deaf and hard of hearing. Recent assessments indicate that Carlos's independent reading skills are significantly below grade level; therefore, he continues to receive reading instruction in a self-contained environment. This class is taught by a teacher of the deaf and hard of hearing, and the reading class has an enrollment of six students. The curriculum being utilized by the teacher is the Direct Instruction *Corrective Reading* series. Carlos's teacher reports that he is making excellent progress in this curriculum. She indicates that, at the beginning of the year, Carlos did not know basic phonics rules or how to apply them to word-reading activities. In addition, she reports that despite Carlos's degree of hearing loss and auditory access to many words, his vocabulary and comprehension skills are also weak. Carlos can also access daily services in the resource classroom for students who are deaf or hard of hearing during his study hall period. Resource services include preteaching vocabulary, previewing reading materials, and reviewing previously taught concepts.

Other

The high school that Carlos attends offers American Sign Language classes for foreign-language credit. Carlos chose this course as his elective for the year. He indicated his desire to improve his expressive sign language skills in order to communicate more readily with his peers who are deaf or hard of hearing and increase his participation in the school's deaf club activities.

CASE STUDY D: DANIELLE

Demographic Information

Danielle is an 11-year-old fifth grader who attends the state school for the deaf. Danielle's parents, Jake and Marcia, both attended the school for the deaf when they were growing up. After graduating from high school, Jake and Marcia attended college at the National Technical Institute for the Deaf in Rochester, New York. Marrying soon after college graduation, the couple returned to the Midwest after the birth of their two children, Danielle and Jordon. Jordon is now 9 years old and enrolled in the fourth grade at the school for the deaf. Jake and Marcia are currently employees of the school for the deaf. Jake is the director of student life, coordinating all services for residential students. Marcia is a classroom assistant in the elementary school. The family lives in the community where the school for the deaf is located, and Danielle and Jordon attend the school under the classification of day students.

Hearing Loss

Given the family history of hearing loss, Danielle's loss was suspected and identified soon after her birth. Audiological exams have consistently indicated a profound, bilateral, sensorineural hearing loss 85/90/95 dB HL at 500, 1000, and 2000 Hz. Danielle has been fitted with hearing aids over the years but, even though she currently owns a pair, she rarely uses them.

Communication System

Danielle and her family use American Sign Language (ASL) to communicate at home. Although Danielle does not vocalize, she does provide appropriate approximations of words on her lips as she signs. The residential school for the deaf that Danielle attends has adopted a bilingual and English as a second language model. Therefore, the primary mode of communication at the school is ASL, although English is also emphasized during instructional activities. In fact, the pairing of ASL and English provides the foundation for many lessons. Concepts and ideas are first presented in ASL to ensure understanding, and then the same concepts are presented in English, typically via print materials.

The school for the deaf recently received a grant to purchase SmartBoards for each classroom. These interactive, electronic whiteboards have allowed teachers increased opportunities to simultaneously present information in ASL and written English. Danielle's parents credit the use of the SmartBoards for her recently increased awareness and interest in printed English and reading. Since using this technology in the classroom, Danielle has been asking to go to the public library to check out books and read magazines. She recently requested a subscription to a teen magazine for her birthday.

Academic History and Present Level of Performance

Danielle has attended the school for the deaf since preschool and has always been a very inquisitive student. Since she was young, Danielle has been interested in learning the appropriate signs or spellings of unknown words. Although Danielle possesses strong skills in communicating and receiving information using ASL, her reading skills lag behind. In fact, results of recent standardized assessments indicate that her word-reading abilities are at approximately the third-grade level and her reading comprehension skills a second-grade level.

Danielle's teacher reports that she can often provide the correct signs for individual words as she reads but experiences difficulty understanding English syntax and answering comprehension questions about what was read. When a passage is presented in ASL and the questions are interpreted, Danielle is readily able to answer questions about topics written at the fifth-grade level. Therefore, it is clear to her teachers and parents that she requires additional instruction in English and gaining meaning from written texts.

Danielle experiences difficulty with many reading comprehension skills and does not appear to monitor her comprehension as she reads. She quickly reads through selections and then asks for assistance from the teacher. In addition to her difficulty with answering written questions previously discussed, Danielle also struggles with recognizing story structure and summarizing main events in the story.

Other

The school for the deaf has a unique art and rhythm program that it offers to elementary students. This program uses a thematic approach in which the children learn dances, customs, and styles of clothing from a variety of countries. For each unit of study, students make clothing items and create art items that are associated with a particular cultural theme. Danielle has excelled in this program over the past two years, and her interest in dance has grown considerably. Beginning in the fall of this year, Danielle has also enrolled in dance lessons at a community dance school. Her parents report that she looks forward to her weekly dance lessons and interacting with her dance teacher and fellow students, all of whom are hearing. Danielle has been working diligently to prepare for her solo dance that she is scheduled to perform during the spring dance recital.

PART 3

INSTRUCTIONAL PRACTICES

C H A P T E R 4

PHONEMIC AWARENESS AND PHONICS

...[D]eep and thorough knowledge of letters, spelling patterns, and words, and of the phonological translations of all three, are of inescapable importance to both skillful reading and its acquisition....Instruction designed to develop children's sensitivity to spelling and their relations to pronunciatiotns should be of paramount importance in the development of reading skills. This is, of course, precisely what is intended in good phonic instruction (Adams, 1990, p. 416).

CHAPTER OBJECTIVES

After completing this chapter, the reader will be able to:

- Describe the National Reading Panel's findings relative to phonemic awareness and phonics instruction

- Explain the findings of studies exploring the efficacy of using phonemic awareness and phonics instruction with students who are deaf or hard of hearing

- Discuss appropriate Individualized Education Plan (IEP) goals and short-term objectives for phonemic awareness and phonics instruction

- Create instructional activities to teach phonemic awareness and phonic skills

- Describe how to incorporate Visual Phonics into instructional activities

INTRODUCTION

According to the findings of the National Reading Panel (2000), balanced and effective reading instruction contains five essential components: (1) phonemic awareness, (2) phonics, (3) fluency, (4) vocabulary, and (5) comprehension. As discussed in Chapter 2, the National Reading Panel (2000) based its recommendations on a review of nearly 100,000 research studies conducted since 1966. Furthermore, a phonetic language such as English requires students, including those who are deaf or hard of hearing, to understand the connection between the phonemes of the language and the graphemes of print. In Chapter 3, the topics of working memory and phonology as they relate to individuals who are deaf or hard of hearing were explored, suggesting that alternative means of acquiring phonology do exist.

In this chapter, the National Reading Panel's (2000) conclusions and suggestions for instruction in the areas of phonemic awareness and phonics are described in greater detail. Studies exploring the efficacy of using phonemic awareness and phonics instruction with students who are deaf or hard of hearing are also reviewed. An overview of several assessments of phonemic awareness and phonic skills is supplied, and sample Individualized Education Program (IEP) goals and objectives for these areas of instruction are provided. Guidelines for sequencing skills evaluations of selected core curricula that include phonemic awareness and phonics instruction as well as sample instructional activities are also included. A detailed description of how to incorporate Visual Phonics into instructional activities is also supplied. In the conclusion, major points are highlighted and directions for future research are discussed.

PHONEMIC AWARENESS

Phonemic awareness is the ability to "notice, think about, and work with the individual sounds in spoken words" (Armbruster, Lehr, & Osborn, 2001, p. 2). Technically, phonemic awareness tasks are not reading tasks but tasks that prepare students to become readers. Phonemic awareness skills involve the ability to recognize that words are made up of phonemes, the smallest units of spoken language, and that phonemes can be manipulated and combined to create spoken words. Simply put, phonemic awareness skills typically involve the manipulation of phonemes in spoken language without the aid of print.

Deciphering the system for distinguishing phonemes is not an easy task. This is in part because spoken language is seamless; there are no breaks when speaking to indicate where one phoneme ends and another begins. The complexity of phonemic awareness is further supported by research that indicates that people who have not developed adequate reading skills typically demonstrate difficulties in performing phonemic awareness tasks (National Reading Panel, 2000). Thus, implementing explicit instruction in phonemic awareness is vital for students to understand the foundation of the alphabetic system and to be able to apply this knowledge to reading and spelling tasks. The National Reading Panel explored eight different types of phoneme manipulation that can be used in instructional activities. Each activity is briefly described in the following section.

Instructional Activities

According to the National Reading Panel (2000), effective phonemic awareness instruction teaches children to manipulate sounds in spoken language. Phonemic awareness activities teach children to notice, think about, and work with the more than 40 phonemes that make up the alphabetic system of the English language. These activities include phoneme (1) isolation, (2) identity, (3) categorization, (4) blending, (5) segmentation, (6) deletion, (7) addition, and (8) substitution (Armbruster et al., 2001).

In phoneme isolation activities, children must recognize and isolate specific phonemes in words. For example, when asked, "What is the first sound in *fan*?," children should respond /f/. Phoneme identity tasks, on the other hand, require students to identify the common phoneme in a set of words. Teachers can prompt this activity by questioning, "What sound is the same in *sing*, *sat*, and *sun*?" In phoneme categorization activities, children are required to recognize the word in a set of three or four that has the *odd* sound. For example, when presented with the list of words *rag*, *run*, and *bat*, children would need to identify *bat* as the word that does not belong. Activities that require children to listen to a sequence of phonemes presented orally and then combine them to create a word are considered to be phoneme blending tasks. For instance, if the teacher asks, "What word is /p/ /a/ /t/?", children should respond with the word *pat* (Armbruster et al., 2001).

Phoneme segmentation tasks require that children recognize, count, and produce individual phonemes in an orally presented word. For example, when asked, "How many sounds

in the word *man*?" the response should be "Three: /m/ /a/ /n/." Children identify the word that remains after a phoneme is removed in phoneme deletion activities. For instance, when the teacher asks, "What word is left when I take the /s/ away from *stop*?" children should reply "Top." In phoneme addition tasks, children must recognize and name the new word produced when a phoneme is added to an existing word. For example, children should recognize that when you add /s/ to the beginning of *park*, the resulting word is *spark*. Finally, in phoneme substitution activities, children substitute one phoneme for another to create a new word. For instance, if the initial word is *fat* and the teacher directs the children to replace /f/ with /s/, then children must realize that the new word is *sat* (Armbruster et al., 2001).

The National Reading Panel (2000) found that the number of phonemic awareness skills as well as which skills should be taught were important considerations. The panel suggested that students' transfer of phonemic awareness skills to reading was strongest when only one or two phonemic awareness skills were focused on at a time. Even though eight different phonemic awareness instructional activities were described in the National Reading Panel (2000) report, the panel indicated that certain tasks were more highly related to reading and spelling tasks. These skills include phoneme blending as it relates to reading and phoneme segmentation as it correlates to spelling.

The National Reading Panel (2000) also made additional comments and recommendations relative to phonemic awareness instruction. First, the panel suggested that essentially all students can benefit from phonemic awareness instruction, including preschoolers, kindergartners, and first graders who are just beginning to read as well as older, less capable readers. In regards to instructional arrangement, the panel reported that small-group instruction may be more effective than individual or whole-group instruction because children can benefit from listening to their classmates' responses as well as from receiving feedback from the teacher. Furthermore, the panel indicated that no more than 20 hours of phonemic awareness instruction was needed over the course of the school year in order to be effective. Finally, the panel pointed out that phonemic awareness skills are taught in order to make phonics instruction easier and more beneficial. Therefore, the panel encouraged teachers to include activities that require children to manipulate phonemes along with letters. Essentially, this pairing of letters with phonemes creates a bridge between phonemic awareness and phonic skills instruction.

PHONICS

The goal of phonics instruction is to help children learn and use the alphabetic principle— the understanding that there is a predictable relationship between letters (graphemes) and sounds (phonemes). Knowledge of these relationships allows children to recognize familiar words accurately and automatically, decode unfamiliar words, and spell words composed of the letter–sound relationships they have been taught. Critics of phonics instruction contend that English spellings are too irregular and children therefore do not benefit from this type of instruction. Proponents of phonics insist that phonics instruction teaches children a system for remembering words and that the alphabetic system is actually a mnemonic device that supports our memory for specific words. Supporters further state that even when a word has an irregular spelling, there is usually a portion of the word that contains some regular letter–sound correspondences (Armbruster et al., 2001). Take the word *said*, for instance. Although the /a/ and /i/ are considered irregular in this word, the

/s/ and /d/ sounds follow a regular pattern of pronunciation. The National Reading Panel (2000) described seven instructional approaches to teaching phonics. Each approach is defined in the following section.

Instructional Approaches

There are several approaches to teaching phonics including (1) analytic phonics, (2) phonics through spelling, (3) embedded phonics, (4) analogy-based phonics, (5) onset-rime phonics, (6) synthetic phonics, and (7) systematic phonics. In an analytic phonics approach, children are taught to first identify a word and then analyze it and determine the letter–sound relations. Using this approach, students are also discouraged from pronouncing phonemes in isolation. A phonics-through-spelling approach relies on children's ability to segment words into individual phonemes and writing the letter that corresponds to that phoneme. Children are taught letter–sound correspondences during the reading of connected text in an embedded phonics approach, whereas in an analogy-based approach, children learn to use parts of word families to identify words with similar parts. Using an onset-rime approach to teaching phonics, children learn to identify the sound of the letter(s) before the first vowel (the onset) and the sound of the remaining part of the word (the rime) in one syllable words. Synthetic phonics focuses on teaching children how to convert letters or letter combinations into sounds and then blending them to form recognizable words, whereas a systematic approach is characterized as teaching a predetermined set of letter–sound relationships in a clearly defined sequence (Armbruster et al., 2001).

The National Reading Panel (2000) concluded that systematic and explicit phonics instruction is more appropriate than nonsystematic phonics instruction or no phonics instruction. In addition to teaching the predetermined letter–sound relationships, this type of instruction also provides children with substantial practice in applying the knowledge they are acquiring to both reading and spelling words. Children are provided with stories containing a large number of words they can decode by using the letter–sound correspondences they have been taught. As discussed in Chapter 2, Chall (1996) referred to these materials as *decodable text*.

To determine whether a beginning reading program could be considered systematic and explicit, the National Reading Panel (2000) supplied several descriptors of nonsystematic approaches. First and foremost, nonsystematic programs do not teach consonant and vowel letter–sound relationships in a prescribed sequence. Instead, nonsystematic approaches typically encourage informal phonics instruction. Nonsystematic phonics approaches often neglect the teaching of vowel sounds even though vowel sounds are considered a critical part of knowing the alphabetic system. Finally, nonsystematic approaches do not provide ample materials or opportunities that foster the application of phonic skills to reading and spelling tasks.

The National Reading Panel (2000) also described additional characteristics of reading programs that would be considered nonsystematic. These include literature-based programs that emphasize reading and writing activities that only teach phonic skills incidentally based on key letters that appear in the text. Basal reading programs that focus on whole-word or meaning-based activities that provide little to no instruction in phonics also fall under the umbrella of nonsystematic approaches. Finally, sight word programs that begin by teaching children approximately 50 to 100 words before they receive instruction in the alphabetic principle are considered nonsystematic.

Based on their findings, the National Reading Panel (2000) offered several additional conclusions regarding systematic and explicit phonics instruction. First, a systematic and explicit phonics approach significantly improves kindergarten and first-grade children's word recognition and spelling skills. Second, systematic and explicit phonics instruction also has a significant impact on children's reading comprehension skills. Third, this approach is proven effective for children from various social and economic levels and is particularly beneficial for children who have difficulty learning to read and those who are at risk of reading failure. Finally, the panel reported that systematic and explicit phonics instruction is most effective when introduced early. The greatest effects were found when instruction began in kindergarten or first grade before students have learned to read independently. The panel also stated that phonics instruction is not an entire reading program for beginning readers. Children should also engage in phonemic awareness activities, reading a variety of texts, as well as writing letters, words, and short stories. Given the importance of explicitly and systematically teaching children phonemic awareness and phonics skills, research studies exploring the use of this approach to teaching beginning reading skills to students who are deaf or hard of hearing are reviewed in the following sections.

PHONEMIC AWARENESS AND PHONICS INSTRUCTION FOR STUDENTS WHO ARE DEAF OR HARD OF HEARING

As discussed in the previous chapters, research evidence suggests that individuals who are deaf or hard of hearing can employ alternative strategies to acquire phonological skills such as phonemic awareness and phonics and apply them to reading tasks. These alternatives include the use of residual hearing, speech reading, and visual cueing systems such as Cued Speech and Visual Phonics. Despite this evidence, there are relatively few intervention studies aimed at integrating phonemic awareness and phonics instruction into beginning reading instruction for students who are deaf or hard of hearing.

Two recently conducted meta-analytic reviews exploring research conducted in the field of reading and deafness substantiate this void (Luckner, Sebald, Cooney, Young, & Goodwin Muir, 2005/2006; Schirmer & McGough, 2005). In their review of the literature, *Teaching Reading to Children Who Are Deaf: Do the Conclusions of the National Reading Panel Apply?*, Schirmer and McGough (2005) examined studies conducted since 1970 that met the following criteria: (1) they identified reading as a variable; (2) they were published in a refereed journal, conference yearbook, or monograph; (3) they focused on the reading development of deaf children between preschool and grade 16; and (4) they used a quantitative or qualitative research design. Schirmer and McGough's search yielded 67 studies; only one was related to the development of phonemic awareness skills among children who are deaf or hard of hearing (Schimmel, Edwards, & Prickett, 1999).

Luckner et al. (2005/2006) used a more stringent standard in their review titled "*An Examination of the Evidence-Based Literacy Research in Deaf Education.*" To be included in this review, studies needed to: (1) be published in a peer-reviewed journal between 1963 and 2003, (2) include study participants who were deaf or hard of hearing, (3) contain a study sample of children and youth between the ages of 3 and 21 years, (4) provide the necessary statistical information to calculate effect size, and (5) employ a control group. Of the 22 studies available for review, none employed phonemic awareness or phonics instruction as an intervention strategy. In addition to the Schimmel, Edwards, and Prickett (1999) study, four additional studies were available that were not included in either of the aforementioned reviews. In the following section, each study is described and the results are reported.

REVIEW OF ADDITIONAL INTERVENTION RESEARCH

In the Schimmel et al. (1999) study, researchers explored the effectiveness of a five-component reading program aimed at improving reading abilities among 48 elementary age students enrolled in a residential school for the deaf. The researchers developed a curriculum addressing phonemic awareness and reading comprehension skills and employed a combination of adapted Dolch word lists, Bridge lists and bridging, and American Sign Language development and language experience stories as intervention strategies. Bridge lists and bridging were described as techniques that were used to teach students to sign English sentences using a conceptually accurate sign system. Students received individual instruction from the five component program two days a week for 20 minutes. The study was conducted over the course of an entire school year, but the actual number of instructional sessions was not reported.

The phonemic awareness component of this reading instructional intervention focused on teaching students 21 consonants, 5 short vowels, and 16 vowel combinations. Although the authors stated that most study participants mastered phonemic awareness by learning to approximate or mouth the consonant and vowel sounds, the method of assessment was not clear.

Furthermore, the researchers indicated that consistent teaching enabled most children to master the sounds, but no description of instructional techniques was included. In addition, the investigators mentioned the role that the acquisition of these skills played in the improvement of students' spelling skills leading one to question whether it was phonics rather than phonemic awareness skills that were addressed through this intervention. The lack of clear descriptions of methods, assessments, and results led Schirmer and McGough (2005) to characterize the study as one "with serious flaws" (p. 89).

The remaining four studies represent those not included in either of the literature reviews previously discussed. The first study explored the efficacy of utilizing a phonics treatment package with middle school students (Trezek & Malmgren, 2005). In this investigation, the first 20 lessons of the Direct Instruction *Corrective Reading—Decoding A* curriculum, a systematic and explicit approach containing both phonemic awareness and phonics instruction, were enhanced for use with students who are deaf or hard of hearing. These enhancements included the use of the Visual Phonics hand cues and a computer program that incorporated a semitransparent *talking head* called *Baldi* and a pictorial glossary. The 23 student participants with hearing losses ranging from mild to profound were randomly assigned to either the treatment or comparison group based on their performance on a curriculum-based measure of the phonemes and words taught through the curriculum.

After 8-weeks of instruction, the students in the treatment group significantly outperformed their comparison group counterparts on tests of the phonemes and words taught as well as a measure of **pseudoword** decoding aimed at exploring the students' ability to generalize the phonic skills acquired. One of the most compelling findings of this study was related to degree of hearing loss and perfor-

mance on test measures. Although degree of hearing loss was correlated with performance on the pretest with the more significant hearing losses related to lower scores on test measures for both students in the treatment and comparison groups, this was not the case with the posttest or generalization test measures for students in the treatment group. In fact, the more significant hearing losses were correlated with higher scores on the generalization test for students in the treatment group. This finding led the authors to conclude that the acquisition and generalization of phonics skills did not appear to be associated with degree of hearing loss, and students with varying degrees of hearing loss could benefit equally from the instruction they received through the phonics treatment package (Trezek & Malmgren, 2005).

Although these findings are extremely encouraging, the computer technology employed in the study is not commercially available, thus making replications of the above study impossible. In a recent investigation, the above study was replicated using only the *Corrective Reading—Decoding A* curriculum supplemented by Visual Phonics hand cues (Trezek, in preparation). Because of the favorable results obtained in the Trezek and Malmgren (2005) study, the program administrator for students who are deaf or hard of hearing would not agree to random assignment of students. Therefore, the pretest, posttest, and generalization scores obtained for 26 students with varying degrees of hearing loss in second through eighth grade were analyzed in this investigation. Results of this inquiry support the findings previously obtained. After an average of 12-weeks of instruction, measures indicated a statistically significant difference between students' performance from pretest to posttest.

The third study explored the use of the Direct Instruction reading curriculum *Reading*

Mastery to address the reading needs of children in kindergarten and first grade (Trezek & Wang, 2006). Similar to the Direct Instruction *Corrective Reading—Decoding A* curriculum utilized in the previously described studies, the *Reading Mastery* program is also characterized as a systematic and explicit curriculum that includes both phonemic awareness and phonics components. However, unlike the *Decoding A* program, which was developed for remedial readers, the *Reading Mastery* program is considered a basal reading program for children in kindergarten and first grade.

In this study, 13 children with severe and profound hearing losses in kindergarten and first grade received instruction from the *Reading Mastery* curriculum over an 8-month period. Similar to the other investigations of this type, instruction students received from the curriculum was enhanced using the Visual Phonics cueing system. Three subtests of the Wechsler Individual Achievement Test-II (WIAT-II)—Word Reading, Pseudoword Decoding, and Reading Comprehension— were administered to students as pretest and posttest measures of reading achievement. Results of these assessments revealed gains on all measures as a result of instruction (Trezek & Wang, 2006). Additional research investigations are currently underway that are aimed at further substantiating the efficacy of employing the Direct Instruction beginning and remedial reading programs supplemented by Visual Phonics with students who are deaf or hard of hearing in various instructional settings, including a residential school for the deaf (Trezek, in preparation).

The final intervention study exploring the use of a systematic and explicit phonemic awareness and phonics-based reading curriculum was conducted with 20 kindergarten and first-grade students over the course of one school year (Trezek, Wang, Woods, Gampp, & Paul, 2007).

The reading curriculum utilized in this study was not a Direct Instruction program but one created by school district personnel in the district where the study took place. However, Visual Phonics was again employed to facilitate the instruction that the students received.

Six subtests of the Dominie Reading and Writing Assessment Portfolio—Sentence Writing Phoneme, Sentence Writing Spelling, Phonemic Awareness Segmentation, Phonemic Awareness Deletion, Phonics Onsets, and Phonics Rimes—were utilized as pre- and posttest assessments of students' progress within the curriculum. The results obtained in this study revealed a statistically significant difference on all six measures of reading from pre- to posttest, indicating the effectiveness of this curricular intervention (Trezek et al., 2007).

Collectively, these four studies represent an initial step in developing a strong line of intervention research exploring the efficacy of phonemic awareness and phonics instruction for students who are deaf or hard of hearing. Results of these inquiries suggest that phonemic awareness and phonics instruction can be modified and supplemented to meet the beginning and remedial reading needs of students who are deaf or hard of hearing. Replication studies currently in progress will serve to further substantiate the findings obtained by Trezek and her colleagues. Two of the studies described here relied on norm-referenced assessments (Trezek & Wang, 2006; Trezek et al., 2007) whereas the remaining two employed a curriculum-based (i.e., criterion-referenced) measure (Trezek & Malmgren, 2005; Trezek, in preparation). Norm-referenced and criterion-referenced tests are excellent tools for assessing students' current level of performance as well as measuring improvements based on instruction. These assessments are described in greater detail in the following section.

ASSESSMENTS OF PHONEMIC AWARENESS AND PHONICS

Formal assessment instruments typically fall into one of two categories: norm-referenced or criterion-referenced. **Norm-referenced assessments** provide a measure of skills and results that are then interpreted relative to a normative sample. Standard scores, percentile ranks, age, and grade-equivalent scores are outcomes of norm-referenced assessments. **Criterion-referenced tests,** on the other hand, are designed to provide a measure of skills that can be interpreted relative to clearly defined domains of learning tasks (i.e., strengths and weaknesses in a specific domain). These assessments usually consist of checklists, rating scales, and rubrics, and results are reported as either a percentage correct or as meeting or exceeding a predetermined proficiency level (Linn & Gronlund, 2000). These two types of assessments can be used in conjunction with one another to gain insights into students' instructional needs.

There are numerous commercially available norm-referenced and criterion-referenced assessments. The Southwest Educational Development Laboratory [SEDL] (2007) has created a database of reading assessments for students in kindergarten through second grade that is available online at http://www.sedl.org. This database provides consumers with access to lists of assessments available to assess a variety of reading skills. Using this database, a search was conducted to determine both norm-referenced

and criterion-referenced assessments recently published that can be utilized to evaluate children's skills in the area of phonemic awareness and phonics. The names of the assessments, copyright, publisher, and Web site for each of the assessments are summarized in Tables 4-1 through 4-4. Using assessments such as these should assist teachers in understanding students' skill levels and in developing appropriate goals and objectives for students. Many of these tests did not employ students who are deaf or hard of hearing as part of the norming sample, which can become a concern in interpreting the scores for this population. However, given our adherence to the qualitative-similarity hypothesis (discussed in Chapter 1) and the findings of the National Reading Panel (2000), we feel that these tests do have relevance for students who are deaf or hard of hearing and can assist teachers in planning appropriate reading instructional goals.

However, we offer a word of caution in using these assessments. It is important for test administrators to understand test tasks and ensure that they are not altered, particularly when using sign language or Visual Phonics to communicate test items. For example, one subtest of the Dynamic Indicators of Basic Early Literacy Skills (DIBELS) (Good & Kaminski, 2007) utilized with kindergarten and first-grade students is phoneme segmentation, which is used to assess the child's ability to segment three- and four-phoneme words. The examiner presents a word orally such as *sat*, and the child must respond by segmenting the

TABLE 4-1 Norm-Referenced Assessments of Phonemic Awareness

Name of Assessment	Copyright	Publisher	Web Site
Comprehensive Test of Phonological Processing (CTOPP)	1999	ProEd	http://www.proedinc.com
Test of Phonological Awareness Skills (TOPAS)	2003	ProEd	http://www.proedinc.com

TABLE 4-2 Criterion-Referenced Assessments of Phonemic Awareness

Name of Assessment	Copyright	Publisher	Web Site
Bader Reading and Language Inventory, 5th edition*	2005	Pearson Education	http://www.prenhall.com/
Basic Reading Inventory, 9th edition*	2005	Kendall/Hunt	http://www.kendallhunt.com
Developmental Reading Assessment K–3, 2nd edition (DRA-2, K-3)*	2006	Celebration Press Pearson Learning Group	http://www.pearsonlearning.com
Dynamic Indicators of Basic Early Literacy Skills, 6th edition (DIBELS-6)*	2005	University of Oregon	http://dibels.uoregon.edu/
Ekwall / Shanker Reading Inventory, 4th edition (ESRI-4)*	2000	Pearson/Allyn & Bacon	http://www.ablongman.com
Phonemic-Awareness Skills Screening (PASS)	2000	ProEd	http://www.proedinc.com
Phonological Awareness Literacy Screening (PALS)*	2005	University of Virginia	http://pals.virginia.edu
Process Assessment of the Learner Test Battery for Reading and Writing (PAL)*	2001	The Psychological Corporation	http://harcourtassessment.com
Standardized Assessment of Phonological Awareness	2006	Professor Garfield	http://www.garfieldu.org
Stieglitz Informal Reading Inventory, 3rd edition*	2002	Pearson/Allyn & Bacon	http://www.ablongman.com
Teaching Beginning Readers: Linking Assessment and Instruction*	2002	Kendall/Hunt	http://www.kendallhunt.com

*Also includes phonics assessments

TABLE 4-3 Norm-Referenced Assessments of Phonics

Name of Assessment	Copyright	Publisher	Web Site
Gray Diagnostic Reading Tests, 2nd edition (GDRT-2)	2004	ProEd	http://www.proedinc.com
Group Reading Assessment and Diagnostic Evaluation (GRADE)	2001	American Guidance Service, Inc.	http://www.agsnet.com
Phonics-Based Reading Test (PRT)	2002	Academic Therapy Publications	http://www.academictherapy.com
Qualitative Reading Inventory, 4th edition (QRI-4)	2006	Pearson/Allyn & Bacon	http://www.ablongman.com
Stanford Achievement Test, 10th edition (SAT-10)	2004	Harcourt Assessment	http://harcourtassessment.com
Test of Oral Reading and Comprehension Skills (TORCS)	2000	Academic Therapy Publications	http://www.academictherapy.com
Test of Silent Word Reading Fluency (TOSWRF)	2004	ProEd	http://www.proedinc.com
Wechsler Individual Achievement Test—Second Edition (WIAT-II)	2005	Harcourt Assessment	http://harcourtassessment.com
Criterion Test of Basic Skills (CTOBS-2)	2002	Academic Therapy Publications	http://www.academictherapy.com
The Critical Reading Inventory	2004	Pearson Education	http://vig.prenhall.com

TABLE 4-4 Criterion-Referenced Assessments of Phonics

Name of Assessment	Copyright	Publisher	Web Site
Criterion Test of Basic Skills (CTOBS-2)	2002	Academic Therapy Publications	http://www.academictherapy.com
The Critical Reading Inventory	2004	Pearson Education	http://vig.prenhall.com
Observation Survey of Early Literacy Achievement, revised second edition	2005	Heinemann	http://www.heinemann.com

word: /s/ /a/ /t/. In this example, if the examiner assessing a child who is deaf or hard of hearing presents the sign for the word *sat* and the child responded with the Visual Phonics cues for /s/ /a/ /t/, then this presentation and response would be consistent with the intended task and the results can then be considered valid.

As you can see from this example, additional tasks also are involved for the child who is deaf or hard of hearing to respond appropriately to this test task. For example, the child would need to know the target word is *sat* rather than *sit*, which is usually designated by using a past tense marker in sign language. Furthermore, this task is made more difficult when the target word does not have a corresponding sign such as *woof* or *ling*. In these cases, the inclination would be to finger spell the word for the child. However, this modification would be analogous to spelling the word orally to a hearing child and then asking her to provide the associated phonemes. As you can see, this veers from the original test task and therefore would invalidate the results obtained. Although the phoneme segmentation task of the DIBELS (Good & Kaminski, 2007) assessment may be invalid measure for some students, several of the other subtests such as Letter-Naming Fluency and Nonsense Word Fluency can be appropriately modified and valid results obtained. Therefore, we encourage test administrators to review each subtest carefully to determine the effects of various administrative procedures.

INSTRUCTIONAL GOALS AND OBJECTIVES

According to the findings of the National Reading Panel (2000), phonemic awareness skills such as blending and segmenting are more closely related to beginning reading skills than are other types of manipulation such as phoneme deletion, addition, and substitution. Furthermore, the panel suggested that children should also be taught to manipulate phonemes by using the letters of the alphabet. As discussed in a previous section of this chapter, the pairing of these activities forms a bridge between phonemic awareness and phonics instruction. Given that phonemic awareness and phonic skills are so closely related to one another, we suggest that teachers write instructional goals and objectives to address these skills simultaneously. In addition, the importance of blending and segmenting has been noted; therefore, these are the key elements teachers should address as part of instruction.

In order to write appropriate goals and objectives, particularly for students' Individualized Education Programs (IEP), teachers need to begin by writing a present level of educational performance for a particular instructional area. The present level of performance should include summative information derived from assessment tools as well as general observations of the student's classroom performance that indicate a need for instruction.

Next, an annual goal is crafted to describe what can reasonably be accomplished given one year of instruction. The short-term objectives or benchmarks are then written to divide the annual goal into discrete instructional components. Most important, goals and short-term objectives must be measurable. The test for measurability would be that multiple evaluators could agree on whether or not the student has achieved the goal or objectives based solely on how the goal has been written (Bateman & Herr, 2006). Additional components of an IEP goal and objectives related to the goal include information on how the goal will be evaluated and measured as well as information on the student's progress toward meeting the annual goal.

A sample annual goal along with short-term objectives to address phonemic awareness and phonics instruction is included in Table 4-5. This sample instructional goal was written to address the beginning reading needs of Aidan, the student who is the subject of Case Study A. For further information regarding Aidan, please refer to the information provided in the case study section of the text.

TABLE 4-5 Annual Goal and Short-Term Objectives for Phonemic Awareness and Phonic Skills

Area of Need: Phonemic Awareness, Phonics, and Spelling

Present Level of Performance:
Aidan's scores on the Letter–Word Identification, Word Attack, Reading Comprehension, and Spelling of Sounds subtests of the Woodcock Johnson Test of Achievement—III indicate performance below average when compared to hearing children of the same age. These results are consistent with his current classroom performance. Although Aidan knows many letter–sound correspondences and can produce the correct Visual Phonics cues to represent the sounds, he has difficulty blending and segmenting sounds and therefore applying this knowledge to reading and spelling activities.

Goal:
Given instruction in letter–sound correspondences, Aidan will be able to read, spell, and define selected phonetically regular words with at least 90% accuracy.

How will progress toward this goal be measured?
Progress notes, teacher observations, word reading, pseudoword reading, and spelling evaluations

Short-term objectives or benchmarks, including criteria for evaluation

- Given a list of 10 phonetically regular words presented orally and with Visual Phonics without the aid of print, Aidan will blend the sounds slowly and then produce the word at a normal rate with at least 90% accuracy.

- Given a list of 10 phonetically regular words containing letter–sound correspondences he has mastered, Aidan will orally blend the sounds with and without Visual Phonics to read the words with at least 90% accuracy.

- Given a list of 10 phonetically regular pseudowords containing letter–sound correspondences he has mastered, Aidan will blend the sounds to read the list of words with at least 90% accuracy.

- When presented with a list of words containing letter–sound correspondences that he has mastered, Aidan will orally segment the words and write the correct spelling with at least 90% accuracy.

- Given a list of 10 phonetically regular words containing letter–sound correspondences he has mastered, Aidan will indicate comprehension of the word by providing the correct sign or description of the word in 9 out of 10 situations.

- Given sentences or short passages containing words which have been previously practiced in isolation, Aidan will read the selection with at least 90% accuracy.

Progress Toward Annual Goal

Date	Progress*	Comments:

*Minimal (M) = anticipate that the goal will not be met by the end of the quarter
Proficient (P) = anticipate that the goal will be met by the end of the quarter
Advanced (A) = anticipate that the goal will be exceeded by the end of the quarter

SEQUENCING PHONEMIC AWARENESS AND PHONICS INSTRUCTION

For teachers to write suitable annual goals and short-term objectives as well as provide effective instruction in phonemic awareness and phonics, it is important to understand how to appropriately sequence and introduce these skills to students. The National Reading Panel (2000) endorsed systematic and explicit phonemic awareness and phonics instructional approaches. To evaluate these key components within a curriculum or to design their own instruction, teachers should keep the following five guidelines in mind: (1) Introduce the most common sound for a letter first, (2) separate sounds that are auditorially similar and letters that are visually similar, (3) introduce the most useful letters first, (4) introduce lowercase letters before uppercase letters, and (5) be aware of the complexity of sound and word types as they are introduced to students (Carnine, Silbert, Kame'enui, & Tarver, 2004).

First, the most common sound for a particular letter is the sound a letter produces when it appears in a short, one-syllable word such as *man* or *dim*. Second, the more similar two letters are, the more likely children will confuse them. Therefore, a carefully sequenced sound introduction list ensures that this confusion is minimized. For example, pairs of sounds such as /f/ and /v/, /k/ and /g/, and /m/ and /n/ are considered auditorially similar, whereas letter pairs such as /b/ and /d/, /m/ and /n/, and /p/ and /q/ are considered visually similar. Therefore, according to Carnine et al. (2004), visually and auditorially similar letters and sounds should be separated

by the introduction of at least three other, dissimilar letters or sounds.

Third, students should be taught more useful letters first. Useful letters are those that appear most often in words and allow students to decode more words earlier. Examples of useful letters include consonants such as *b, c, d, f, g, h, k, l, m, n, p, r, s, t,* and vowel sounds. The letters *j, q, z, y, x, v,* and *w* are considered less useful. Fourth, lowercase letters should be taught before uppercase letters because the majority of letters students encounter in words are lowercase. When an uppercase letter is formed in a similar manner to the lowercase letter (e.g., *Cc, Oo, Ss*), the upper- and lowercases can be introduced simultaneously, whereas visually dissimilar pairs (*Aa, Dd, Hh*) should be avoided (Carnine et al., 2004).

Finally, teachers should be aware of the complexity of sound and word types before deciding on a sequence of instruction. Continuous sounds are those that can be held for several seconds (e.g., /f/, /l/, /m/) whereas stop sounds can be said for only an instant (e.g., /b/, /c/, /d/); therefore, continuous sounds are initially easier for children to produce. In addition to the difficulty of individual sounds, teachers must also be aware of the complexity of word types based on vowel (V) and consonant (C) patterns. For example, words containing a V-C or C-V-C pattern are less difficult than those containing a C-C-V-C-C pattern. As each new pattern of words is introduced, teachers should utilize continuous sounds first and then make the transition to words of the same pattern that include stop sounds (Carnine et al., 2004). These principles of effective sound and letter sequencing ensure student success and, therefore, should be used to guide instruction.

PHONEMIC AWARENESS AND PHONICS INSTRUCTION IN CORE READING CURRICULA

As previously noted, the majority of children require direct instruction in phonemic awareness and phonics in order to become successful readers. There are many reading curriculums available to address students' needs in these skill areas; the most successful include skill instruction within the broader content of a balanced reading program. The American Federation of Teachers [AFT] recognizes the importance of identifying a strong, core reading curriculum that focus on all five areas of instruction identified by the National Reading Panel (2000). In order to evaluate the strengths and weaknesses of commercially available curricula, the AFT recommends the use of *A Consumer's Guide to Evaluating a Core Reading Program, Grades K–3: A Critical Elements Analysis*, which is available at http://reading.uoregon.edu.

This consumer guide created by Simmons and Kame'enui (2003) specifies criteria for reviewing critical elements of reading instruction by grade level. For example, in evaluating curricula created for kindergarten students, the following areas of instruction are assessed: (1) phonological and phonemic awareness, (2) letter–sound association, (3) decoding, (4) irregular words, (5) vocabulary, and (6) listening comprehension. Curricula for first-grade students evaluate instruction in the following areas: (1) phonemic awareness, (2) phonics and word analysis, (3) irregular words, (4) text reading and fluency, (5) vocabulary, and (6) reading comprehension. These criteria are clearly substantiated by the theoretical foundations of reading development put forth by Chall (1996) and other cognitive–interactive theorists and is also aligned with the findings of the National Reading Panel (2000).

Using the charts provided by these authors (Simmons & Kame'enui, 2003), kindergarten through third-grade curricula can be rated as to whether the instructional intervention consistently meets, partially meets, or does not satisfy the designated criterion for each instructional element. The authors also specify the type of review that will best analyze each element of instruction. These review types include sections titled *within a sequence of lessons* in which a skill is analyzed within a particular lesson or series of two to three lessons, *scope and sequence* whereby the scope and sequence for the curriculum is examined, and *skill trace*, which requires an examination of a series of 10 consecutive lessons (Simmons & Kame'enui, 2003).

Recently, the Oregon Reading First Center (2004) applied the Simmons and Kame'enui (2003) evaluation criteria to provide a thorough and objective analysis of comprehensive reading programs to assist schools in identifying effective kindergarten through third-grade-level reading curricula. The curricula reviewed were those submitted by publishers that met the Oregon state standards to be considered a comprehensive, beginning reading program. A summary of this review of nine different beginning reading programs—*Harcourt, Houghton Mifflin, Macmillian/McGraw-Hill, Open Court, Reading Mastery, Rigby Literacy, Scott Foresman, Success for All* and *Wright Group*—is available online at http://reading. uoregon.edu.

For the purposes of this chapter, the summary data for the high-priority skill items of phonemic awareness and phonics for kindergarten through third grade were reviewed. Phonemic awareness instruction was evaluated for both the kindergarten and first-grade levels. At the kindergarten level, curricula with the highest percentage ratings included *Reading Mastery* (95%), *Houghton Mifflin* and

Macmillian/McGraw-Hill (85%), and *Open Court* and *Harcourt* (80%). At the first-grade level, programs with the highest ratings for the high-priority skill of phonemic awareness were *Harcourt*, *Houghton Mifflin* and *Reading Mastery* (100%), *Macmillian/McGraw-Hill*, *Open Court*, *Scott Foresman*, and *Success for All* (75%).

Phonics was considered an essential element of instruction for students in kindergarten through third grade. Programs with the highest ratings were *Success for All* (97%), *Macmillian/McGraw-Hill* (89%), *Reading Mastery* (86%), *Harcourt* (75%), and *Scott Foresman* (72%) at the kindergarten level; *Reading Mastery* and *Success for All* (93%), *Open Court* (89%), *Harcourt* (86%), and *Houghton Mifflin* (82%) at the first-grade level; *Houghton Mifflin* (88%), *Reading Mastery* (86%), *Scott Foresman* (81%), *Harcourt* (75%), and *Wright Group* (63%) at the second-grade level; and *Harcourt* and *Reading Mastery* (100%), *Houghton Mifflin* (88%), and *Rigby* and *Scott Foresman* (75%) at the third-grade level. We encourage readers to explore the aforementioned curricula or evaluate curricula not included in this review in order to identify effective, comprehensive, beginning reading curricula to implement with students who are deaf or hard of hearing.

In addition to published reading curricula, many print and online resources are available to provide teachers with ideas for teaching and reinforcing phonemic awareness and phonics skills in entertaining and engaging ways. A selected list of teacher resources and children's books that can be utilized to teach and reinforce phonemic awareness and phonics skills are included at the end of this chapter. Teachers can also create their own activities based on the guidelines provided in the previous section. Several teacher-created activities are described in the following sections.

Phonemic Awareness Instructional Activities

Phonemic awareness activities can be developed to focus on several of the skills outlined by the National Reading Panel (2000) such as phoneme isolation, identity, categorization, blending, segmentation, deletion, addition, and substitution. In fact, activities can be created that focus on one or more of these skills and incorporate the use of letters, which was also recommended by the National Reading Panel. The following activities demonstrate how the above skills can be incorporated into daily instructional activities for children.

- *Initial Sound Book:* Each child in the class is supplied with a piece of construction paper and assigned a specific phoneme. On the back of the paper, the child writes her assigned letter. Using magazines, each child locates, cuts out, and pastes pictures that have her phoneme in the initial sound position on the front of the paper. When completed, each child can present her collage to the class. The teacher can compile the students' papers and form an *Initial Sound Book* for the classroom library. Using the pages in the book, the teacher can lead the students through phoneme identification, blending, and segmenting activities. For example, when viewing the collage for the /m/ sound, the teacher may ask, "What is the first sound of all the pictures on this page? We have *map*, *magazine*, *mop*, *mother*, *mouse*, and *man*. All these items begin with what sound? [phoneme identity]. Yes, /mmm/. Let's see if you are correct." The teacher can then turn the page and reveal the letter on the back of the page. "You were right! What letter makes the sound /mmm/? Yes, *m*. The letter *m* makes the sound /mmm/. Now let's look back at the pictures. We have *man*, *map*, and *mop*. I'll say the sounds in *man* slowly, then I'll say the word. Listen. /mmm/ /aaa/ /nnn/. *Man*. Can you say the sounds in *man* slowly?" [phoneme blending]. The teacher can then repeat this task with the remaining words. These words were specifically targeted because they are phonetically regular words with a C-V-C pattern. In addition, these words contain mostly continuous sounds. When a stop sound is included in the word, it occurs at the end, which will make the blending of sounds easier for the children. "Now let's try counting the sounds in those words [phoneme segmentation]. *Man*. What's the first sound? Next sound? Next sound? How many sounds in *man*? Yes, three. There are three sounds in the word *man*: /mmm/ /aaa/ /nnn/." This task can also be repeated with the targeted words. To modify this activity, struggling students can be partnered with more advanced students to collaborate on the page for the *Initial Sound Book*. To extend this activity, another book can be created to focus on the ending sound of words.

- *Fishing for Sounds:* To plan for this activity, use brightly colored paper cut in the shape of fish and attach a small paper clip to each. Write a different letter or letter combination on each fish. The fish are then placed upside down so that the letters are not visible to the students. Using a fishing pole (a stick with a string and magnet attached), each child takes a turn fishing for a sound. Once the sound has been caught, the teacher can lead the group through a series of activities such as naming words that begin or end with that sound. Phoneme blending, segmentation, deletion, addition, or substitution activities can also be incorporated.

- Write letters on large sheets of paper and place them on the ground. Students toss a bean bag on a letter, say the sound, and think of a word that begins with that sound. Point values can be assigned to each letter, and teams of students can play this game to see which team earns the most points.

- Create a set of cards with one letter on each card. Place the cards in the center of the circle and sing the song "Where is the /mmm/? Where is the /mmm/? /mmmmmm/. Where is the /mmm/?" to the tune of *Farmer in the Dell*. This activity can be used to review previously taught sounds.

- Ask students to sit in a circle. One student chooses a sound written on a small piece of folded paper from a jar and says the sound. Going around the circle, children will say a word that begins or contains the sound. The challenge is to see if they can complete the circle with one sound.

As with the first two examples provided, teachers can extend these activities to include a variety of phonemic awareness tasks to foster skill development.

Phonics Instructional Activities

Following a similar manner of instruction as the phonemic awareness tasks described above, teachers can use the following activities to teach and reinforce the phonic skills children are learning, focusing on target skills such as letter–sound correspondences, phoneme blending, segmenting, addition, deletion, and so on.

- Using a dry erase board, the teacher can start by writing a word such as *sat*. Students then pass the board around the circle, substituting the beginning or ending sound to create different words (i.e., *fat*, *fan, man, mat*, etc.). The student who cannot think of a new word is *out*.

- Replicate a computer keyboard on a large piece of butcher paper. The teacher can either direct this activity or have children work as partners to complete this task in a learning center. The game begins by drawing a card that contains a word that has been previously introduced and practiced. The teacher or partner reads the word such as a *mat* to the student. The student must then hop to each individual letter while saying the sounds /mmm/ /aaa/ /t/ and then hop to the space bar and say the whole word *mat*. This activity is good for students who benefit from movement and gross motor activities.

- A simple bingo game is an excellent way to review and reinforce previously taught letter–sound relationships.

- *Word Ladder:* Draw a word ladder on the board. Write a word at the top of the ladder and a different word at the bottom of the ladder. Explain to the students that their goal is to change the word at the top of the ladder to the word at the bottom by manipulating one letter at a time. The following is an example of a word ladder:

    map

    mop

    top

    tip

    sip

    sit

- *Swat*: Write the sounds, sound combinations, or words you wish to review randomly on the board and divide the class into two teams. One player from each team goes to the board with a fly swatter, and the teacher produces a sound or the sounds in a particular word. When the teacher says, *Go*, the students must find the correct corresponding letter or word. The first student to swat the word earns a point for her team.

INCORPORATING VISUAL PHONICS INTO INSTRUCTIONAL ACTIVITIES

To make these phonemic awareness and phonics activities accessible and effective for students who are deaf or hard of hearing, Visual Phonics can be incorporated into instructional activities. As discussed in Chapter 3, Visual Phonics is a system of 46 hand cues and corresponding written symbols used in conjunction with speech and/or speech reading. This multisensory cueing system was designed to represent the phonemes of English in a visual, tactile, kinesthetic manner. Because Visual Phonics is an instructional tool and not a communication system, it can be incorporated into instruction that uses any communication methodology (e.g., oralism, Signed English, American Sign Language, etc.). If a school program has adopted Cued Speech as its communication methodology, this system can also be used to convey the necessary phonemic information in these activities to students.

To illustrate how to incorporate Visual Phonics into instructional activities, we will use the *Initial Sound Book* activity described above as an example. During instructional activities, Visual Phonics is utilized any time the teacher or student makes reference to a sound. Speech or sign language can then be used to convey the other portions of the intended message. When using Visual Phonics in conjunction with speech or sign language, using a body shift is often helpful. For example, when referring to a sound using Visual Phonics, the teacher can lean to the right; when referring to a letter name or word, the teacher can lean to the left. This body shift reinforces to students the difference between the representation of a sound versus a letter or word.

As part of the sample instructional activity described above, the teacher used the statement, "We have *man*, *map,* and *mop*. I'll say the sounds in *man* slowly, then I'll say the word. Listen. /mmm/ /aaa/ /nnn/. Man." The teacher would incorporate Visual Phonics in the following manner. "We have *man*, *map*, and *mop*. I'll say the sounds in *man* slowly, then I'll say the word. Listen. [Represented with sign language, leaning left.] /mmm/ /aaa/ /nnn/ [represented with Visual Phonics, leaning right]. *Man*" [represented with sign language, leaning left].

The same presentation method is used when incorporating finger spelling into instructional activities. For example, when the teacher says, "The letter *m* makes the sound /mmm/," it would be represented in the following manner: "The letter [represented with sign language, leaning left] *m* [represented with finger spelling, leaning left] makes the sound [represented with sign language, leaning left] /mmm/" [represented with Visual Phonics, leaning right].

Depending on the age and skill level of the students as well as the desired outcome of the activity, the teacher may also choose to simply reinforce the initial sound in words by providing the Visual Phonics cue for the initial sound and pairing it with the sign for the subsequent word. For example, in the statement "We have *map*, *magazine*, *mop*, *mother*, *mouse*, and *man*" the teacher could reinforce the initial sound by representing this sentence as "We have [represented with sign language, leaning left] /mmm/ [represented with Visual Phonics, leaning right] *map*, [represented with sign language, leaning left], /mmm/ [represented with

Visual Phonics, leaning right], *magazine* [represented with sign language, leaning left], /mmm/ [represented with Visual Phonics, leaning right], *mop*, [represented with sign language, leaning left]," and so on.

In activities that require the student to produce sounds and words, a combination of Visual Phonics and sign language is also used. For example, if the teacher asks, "Can you say the sounds in *man* slowly?" the response expected from the students would be the Visual Phonics hand cues and associated vocalization or mouth movements for the sounds /mmm/ /aaa/ /nnn/.

Recently published intervention studies exploring the use of systematic and explicit phonemic awareness and phonics instruction with students who are deaf or hard of hearing have relied primarily on scripted instructional programs supplemented by Visual Phonics (Trezek & Malmgren, 2005; Trezek & Wang, 2006; Trezek et al., 2007). In these curricular interventions, students are required to produce the sounds in the words slowly, sound by sound, without stopping between the sounds; produce the word at a normal rate; and then identify the word during word reading tasks. When the Direct Instruction *Reading Mastery* (Trezek & Wang, 2006) and *Corrective Reading—Decoding A* (Trezek & Malmgren, 2005) curricula were employed in these interventions, this word-reading procedure is utilized throughout the program as students learn to decode new words. In this activity, the teacher is instructed to use the following directives to prompt the students' responses: "Sound it out. Get ready. Again, get ready. Say it fast. What word?"

To modify the instructional procedure to be more conducive for signing and thus more conceptually accurate, the teacher script is slightly altered. Instead of using the terminology "Sound it out," the teacher of the deaf or hard of hearing can sign or say, "Say the sounds." Although the expressions "Say it fast" and "What word?" are not changed, a very specific response is required of the students. Trezek has coined her four-step teaching and response procedure *chaining*.

In the first step of the chaining procedure, the students are prompted to "Say the sounds." At this time, the students are expected to provide the correct Visual Phonics cues and mouth movements that correspond to the model the teacher is providing or to the letters being shown. If the student is using vocalization while producing the cues, the correct vocal sensation (voiced versus unvoiced) should also be produced. This task is then repeated in the second step of the chaining procedure when the teacher prompts the students using the phrase "Again, say the sounds." When prompted to "Say it fast," the third step in the process, the student provides only the mouth movements and possibly the associated vocal response. During this phase of the chaining procedure, the Visual Phonics cues are not employed because it has been found that students have difficulty producing the hand cues while retaining the critical points of articulation, the key element for students to retain. Finally, in the fourth stage of Trezek's chaining procedure, students produce the corresponding sign for or finger spell the representation of the resulting word when the teacher says, "What word?"

As with the instructional activity illustrated previously, body shifting also plays an important role in the four-step chaining procedure. When asking the student to "Say the sounds," the instructor leans right and maintains that position when prompting the second portion of the procedure saying, "Again, say the sounds." When directing the students to "Say it fast," the teacher's body is placed in the neutral or center sign position. When prompting the students with the directive "What word?" the teacher shifts her body to the left. This body-

shifting procedure illustrates the *chaining* and thereby the connection between the Visual Phonics hand cues, the mouth movements and vocal sensations, and, in the end, the resulting signed representation of the word. This procedure is also a helpful tool to convey the difference between English and American Sign Language (ASL) when ASL is the communication system being employed to instruct students. In addition, because this body shift is perceived by the student viewing the cues in a left-to-right orientation, this four-step chaining procedure also serves to reinforce the left-to-right orientation of print reading.

REMEDIAL INSTRUCTION

As discussed in Chapter 2, phonemic awareness and phonics skills begin developing in the preschool years and, for the most part, are fully developed by the end of second grade or Chall's (1996) Stage 2. Because reading skills develop following a hierarchical and interactive progression, it is difficult to progress to the next stage of development if the necessary prerequisite skills are not acquired. We believe this is the case for the majority of students who are deaf or hard of hearing. Traditionally, reading instruction for this population of students has not focused on the development of phonemic awareness and phonics skills as outlined in Chall's Stages 0 through 2; therefore, many students are unable to progress to using reading as a tool for learning. The lack of attention focused on phonemic awareness and phonics skills among readers who are deaf or hard of hearing also contributes to the fourth-grade reading ceiling discussed in Chapter 1. This phenomenon will be discussed further in the subsequent chapters focusing on fluency, vocabulary, and comprehension instruction.

According to Chall (1996), students who lack the necessary prerequisite skills to progress through the stages of reading development must be provided with instruction in the areas lacking. This will probably be the case for many readers who are deaf or hard of hearing beyond the second-grade level. As with young beginning readers, these older remedial readers will require systematic and explicit instruction in phonemic awareness and phonics. However, many of the available curricula for developing these critical skills are geared toward the age and developmental levels of the kindergarten or first-grade students. Therefore, one of the challenges is to identify age-appropriate curricular interventions for these students that will teach the necessary skills at a pace that will allow them to master these skills quickly and effectively.

In 1999, the AFT published *Building on the Best Learning from What Works: Five Promising Remedial Reading Intervention Programs*. Although five programs were recommended, only three of the five programs specifically addressed the remedial reading needs of students in the second and higher grades: (1) Direct Instruction *Corrective Reading*, (2) Exemplary Center for Reading Instruction (ECRI), and (3) Lindamood-Bell. This led the AFT to also include these programs in its publication *Improving Low Performing High Schools* (1999.). We again encourage readers to explore these as well as other remedial reading curricular options and adapt them for use with remedial readers who are deaf or hard of hearing.

CONCLUSION

This chapter focused on the importance of phonemic awareness and phonics instruction for children and adolescents who are deaf or hard of hearing. The discussion of these two areas was guided by the recommendations of the National Reading Panel (2000) and by a synthesis of the available research individuals who are deaf or hard of hearing. This chapter and the preceding Chapter 3 have demonstrated the importance of phonology and the use of a phonological code in the development of both general English-language and reading skills. In addition, it seems to be possible for children with severe to profound hearing losses to have access to phonology via alternative means such as Cued Speech/Language and Visual Phonics.

An overall level of phonological awareness seems to be necessary before children can proceed to phonemic awareness and, subsequently, to the use of phonics skills. Phonological awareness refers to a general understanding or appreciation of the sounds of speech, not their meanings. Phonemic awareness means that a child understands that a word can be divided into a sequence of phonemes (i.e., consonants and vowels) and acquires the skills to manipulate the phonemes. *Phonics* refers to instruction on the manner in which the sounds of speech are represented by letters and spellings.

As shown in this chapter, there is a strong relationship between children's ability to read and their ability to segment words into phonemes, especially in the early grades. Explicit, systematic instructional activities for both phonemic awareness and phonics are important for developing an adequate understanding of the alphabetic principle. With respect to a phonetic language such as English, this principle entails the relationships between sounds and their corresponding representations in print—that is, letters.

CHAPTER SUMMARY

- The National Reading Panel delineated eight different types of phoneme manipulation that can be used in instructional

activities: (1) isolation, (2) identity,
(3) categorization, (4) blending,
(5) segmentation, (6) deletion,
(7) addition, and (8) substitution.

- The approaches to teaching phonics
  include (1) analytic phonics, (2) phonics
  through spelling, (3) embedded phonics,
  (4) analogy-based phonics, (5) onset-rime
  phonics, (6) synthetic phonics, and
  (7) systematic phonics.

- Two meta-analytic reviews on students
  who are deaf or hard of hearing revealed
  few investigations on phonemic awareness and phonics instruction. Obviously,
  there is a need for more intervention
  studies in these areas. The work of Trezek
  and her collaborators represents an initial
  step in developing a strong line of intervention research exploring the efficacy
  of phonemic awareness and phonics
  instruction for students who are deaf or
  hard of hearing.

- For teachers to write suitable annual
  goals and short-term objectives as well
  as provide effective instruction in

phonemic awareness and phonics, it is
important to understand how to appropriately sequence and introduce these
skills to students. Students who have not
mastered phonemic awareness and
phonics skills by the end of second grade
may require remedial instruction. It is
imperative to identify age-appropriate
curricula and methods for teaching
these skills as quickly and effectively as
possible.

- The *chaining* procedure developed by
  Trezek is an effective means of incorporating both Visual Phonics and sign
  language into phonemic awareness and
  phonics instructional activities. This chaining procedure communicates the connection between the Visual Phonics hand cues,
  mouth movements and vocalizations, and
  the resulting sign for target words while
  simultaneously illustrating the difference
  between English and ASL and reinforcing
  the left-to-right orientation of reading
  print.

REVIEW QUESTIONS

1. The National Reading Panel suggested
   that systematic and explicit instruction in
   phonemic awareness and phonics produces the best results. What are the key
   features of this type of instruction?

2. What are the general conclusions of
   the studies exploring the efficacy of
   phonemic awareness and phonics
   instruction for students who are deaf
   or hard of hearing?

3. What are the differences between
   norm-referenced and criterion-referenced
   assessments? How can they be used
   together to gain insight into students'
   instructional needs?

4. Briefly describe the five guidelines
   for sequencing phonemic awareness
   and phonics instruction.

REFLECTIVE QUESTIONS

1. In this chapter, the authors provide a description of Trezek's *chaining* procedure, which is utilized during phonics instruction for students who are deaf or hard of hearing. Using the sample provided in the chapter, write a script that illustrates how you would use the *chaining* procedure to teach a specific phonics activity to a group of first-grade students who are deaf or hard of hearing.

2. According to Chall's stage theory, students who have not acquired fluency in phonemic awareness and phonic skills by third grade will experience great difficulty using reading as a tool for learning. How would you address the instructional needs of older children who continue to struggle with phonemic awareness and phonic skills? Create two activities to address the needs of struggling, remedial readers who are deaf or hard of hearing.

APPLICATION EXERCISES

1. Using the examples provided in this chapter as your guide, create two instructional activities to teach phonemic awareness skills and two instructional activities to teach phonic skills that address the instructional goals and objectives outlined for Aidan, the subject of Case Study A.

2. Write a present level of performance, an annual goal, and at least three short-term objectives to address the phonemic awareness and phonics needs of Brianna, the subject of Case Study B.

SUGGESTED READINGS AND RESOURCES

Readings

Blevins, W. (1997). *Phonemic awareness activities for early reading success* (grades k-2). New York: Scholastic Professional Books.

Blevins, W. (2001). *Teaching phonics and word study in the intermediate grades: A complete sourcebook*. New York: Scholastic Inc.

Leber, N. J. (2003). *Picture sorting for phonemic awareness*. New York: Scholastic Professional Books.

McCormick, C. E., Throneburg, R. N., & Smitely, J. M. (2002). *A sound start: Phonemic awareness lessons for reading success*. New York: Guilford Press.

Ramsey, M. (1999). *Phonic games kids can't resist* (grades K-2). New York: Scholastic Professional Books.

Sanders, M. I. (2001). *Twenty-five read and write mini-books that teach word families*. New York: Scholastic Professional Books.

Scott, V. G. (2005). *Phonemic awareness: Ready-to-use lesson activities and games*. Minnetonka, MN: Peytral Publications.

Wagstaff, J. (2001). *Irresistible sound matching sheets and lessons that build phonemic awareness.* New York: Scholastic Professional Books.

Resources

Carl's Corner
http://www.carlscorner.us/

Free Phonics Worksheets
http://www.free-phonics-worksheets.com/

LessonPlansPage.com
http://www.lessonplanspage.com/

Phonicsworld.com
http://www.phonicsworld.com/

Read, Write, Think
http://www.readwritethink.org/

Starfall.com
http://www.starfall.com/

References

Adams, M. (1990). *Beginning to read: Thinking and learning about print.* Cambridge: MIT Press.

American Federation of Teachers (1999). *Improving Low Performing High Schools.* Retrieved December 15, 2007, from http://www.aft.org/pubs-reports/downloads/teachers/lphs.pdf.

Armbruster, B. B., Lehr, F., & Osborn, J. (2001). *Put reading first: The research building blocks for teaching children to read kindergarten through grade three.* Jessup, MD: National Institute for Literacy.

Bateman, B. D., & Herr, C. M. (2006). *Writing measurable IEP goals and objectives.* Verona, WI: Attainment.

Carnine, D. W., Silbert, J., Kame'enui, E. J., & Tarver, S. G. (2004). *Direct instruction reading.* (4th ed.). Upper Saddle River, NJ: Pearson Education.

Chall, J. S. (1996). *Stages of reading development.* (2nd ed.). New York: McGraw-Hill.

Good, R. H., & Kaminski, R. A. (Eds.). (2007). *Dynamic indicators of basic early literacy skills* (6th ed.). Eugene, OR: Institute for the Development of Educational Achievement. Available: http://dibels.uoregon.edu/.

Linn, R. L., & Gronlund, N. E. (2000). *Measurement and assessment in teaching* (8th ed.). Upper Saddle River, NJ: Prentice Hall.

Luckner, J. L., Sebald, A. N., Cooney, J., Young, J., & Goodwin Muir, S. (2005/2006). An examination of the evidence-based literacy research in deaf education. *American Annals of the Deaf, 150* (5), 443–456.

National Reading Panel. (2000). *Report of the National Reading Panel: Teaching children to read—An evidence-based assessment of the scientific research literature on reading and its implications for reading instruction.* Jessup, MD: National Institute for Literacy at EDPubs.

Oregon Reading First Center. (2004). *Review of Comprehensive Reading Programs.* Retrieved October 21, 2007, from http://reading.uoregon.edu/curricula/intro_summ_review_3-04.pdf.

Schirmer, B. R., & McGough, S. M. (2005). Teaching reading to children who are deaf: Do the conclusions of the National Reading Panel apply? *Review of Educational Research, 75* (1), 83–117.

Schimmel, C. S., Edwards, S. G., & Prickett, H. T. (1999). Reading? . . . Pah! (I got it!):

Innovative reading techniques for successful deaf readers. *American Annals of the Deaf, 144* (4), 298–308.

Simmons, D.C. & Kame'enui, E. J. (2003). *A Consumer's Guide to Evaluating a Core Reading Program, Grades K-3: A Critical Elements Analysis.* Retrieved October 21, 2007 from http://teacher.scholastic.com/products/fundingconnection/pdf/Kameenui_GR_Blue.pdf

Southwest Educational Development Laboratory. (2007). *Reading assessment database.* Retrieved March 3, 2007, from http://www.sedl.org/reading/rad/database.html.

Trezek, B. J. (in preparation). *Phonics instruction for students who are deaf or hard of hearing.* Manuscript in preparation.

Trezek, B. J., & Malmgren, K. W. (2005). The efficacy of utilizing a phonics treatment package with middle school deaf and hard-of-hearing students. *Journal of Deaf Studies and Deaf Education, 3,* 257–271.

Trezek, B. J., & Wang, Y. (2006). Implications of utilizing a phonics-based reading curriculum with children who are deaf or hard of hearing. *Journal of Deaf Studies and Deaf Education, 11,* 202–213.

Trezek, B. J., Wang, Y., Woods, D. G., Gampp, T. L., & Paul, P. (2007). Using Visual Phonics to supplement beginning reading instruction for students who are deaf or hard of hearing. *Journal of Deaf Studies and Deaf Education, 12* (3), 373–384.

CHAPTER 5

FLUENCY

Because the ability to obtain meaning from print depends so strongly on the development of word recognition accuracy and reading fluency, both of the latter should be regularly assessed in the classroom, permitting timely and effective instructional response when difficulty or delay is apparent (Snow, Burns & Griffin, 1998, p. 7).

CHAPTER OBJECTIVES

After completing this chapter, the reader will be able to:

- Describe the National Reading Panel's findings relative to fluency instruction
- Discuss the additional research that has been conducted on repeated readings
- Explain the research exploring the efficacy of fluency instruction with students who are deaf or hard of hearing
- Delineate the questions surrounding implementing reading fluency interventions with students who are deaf or hard of hearing
- Discuss appropriate Individualized Education Program (IEP) goals and short-term objectives for reading fluency instruction
- Create instructional activities to foster fluent reading

INTRODUCTION

*A*s discussed in Chapter 2, developing reading fluency provides a critical bridge between word reading and text comprehension. Developing automatic decoding skills ensures that readers can recognize most words automatically; therefore, cognitive attention can shift from decoding words to focusing on meaning. Chall (1996) and other cognitive scholars emphasized the importance of developing automaticity in decoding words in order for readers to transition from learning to read to reading to learn. The importance of developing reading fluency was also confirmed by the findings of the National Reading Panel (2000).

In this chapter, the National Reading Panel's (2000) conclusions and suggestions for instruction in the area of reading fluency are described in greater detail. Additional research on using repeated readings to improve reading fluency is also presented, and studies exploring the efficacy of implementing fluency instruction with students who are deaf or hard of hearing are reviewed. Guidelines for implementing fluency instruction with students who are deaf or hard of hearing are discussed, and an overview of several assessments of fluency is supplied. A sample Individualized Education Program (IEP) goal and objectives to address reading fluency needs are also provided. Evaluations of selected core curricula that include fluency instruction as well as sample fluency instructional activities are also included. In the chapter summary, major points are highlighted and directions for future research are discussed.

FLUENCY

The National Reading Panel (2000) defined fluency as the ability to read a text accurately and quickly with proper expression. As previously mentioned, Chall (1996) also called for the development of automaticity in Stage 2. *Automaticity* generally refers to the ability to read words, typically in isolation, with accuracy and speed. Although the ability to read words in isolation is necessary to achieve reading fluency, automaticity alone is not sufficient for the development of fluency. Some children are able to recognize words in isolation but are unable to read the same words in connected text. Children who are fluent readers read with accuracy, speed, and expression. Thus, the development and assessment of fluency skills should focus on all three areas.

When reading silently, fluent readers recognize words automatically and are able to group words together in order to gain meaning from what they read. When reading orally, fluent readers read as if they are speaking: effortlessly and with proper expression. These readers also pause at appropriate times and use punctuation to determine when to change emphasis and tone (National Reading Panel, 2000). In contrast, readers who are unable to read fluently read slowly, word by word, and their oral reading is considered "chopping and plodding" (Armbruster, Lehr, & Osborn, 2001, p. 22). It is also important to note that fluency can vary, depending on the reader's familiarity with the words in the text, text type, and the amount of practice they have had with reading the text. For example, a student who is reading a text about an unfamiliar, complex topic such as statistics may need to spend more time and energy on decoding difficult terms or focusing on meaning; as a result, fluency may be reduced.

In their extensive review of the literature, the National Reading Panel (2000) explored two major methods typically used to promote fluent reading. The first method examined was independent silent reading in which students read on their own with minimal guidance or feedback from the teacher. Drop Everything and Read (DEAR) and Silent Sustained Reading (SSR) are common educational practices that employ independent silent reading. Although studies have attempted to discover correlations between independent silent reading and fluency, the National Reading Panel (2000) found no evidence to support the effectiveness of silent reading practices for developing fluency.

The second approach explored by the National Reading Panel (2000)— guided, repeated oral reading— proved more promising than independent silent reading. According to the research, fluency can be developed by having students engage in repeated oral reading using a variety of strategies such as student–adult, choral, tape-assisted, and partner reading as well as through readers' theater activities. Each instructional activity is described in further detail below.

Repeated Reading Instructional Strategies

All five of the recommended instructional strategies for promoting fluent reading incorporate repeated readings. Generally speaking, students require between three and five repetitions to achieve improved fluency (National Reading Panel, 2000). Using the *student–adult instructional strategy*, the student reads with an adult in a one-on-one instructional arrangement. Instruction begins with the adult reading the passage to model accurate and expressive reading at an appropriate rate. Following the adult model, the student reads the same passage, and feedback concerning rate, accuracy, and expression is provided. In the second strategy, *choral reading*, a student or group of students read in unison with the teacher or another fluent reader. The third strategy, *tape-assisted reading*, allows a student to read along while listening to an audiotaped version of the text. During the first presentation of the reading, the student listens to the tape, pointing to each word of the text as the reader reads. For the second repetition of the reading, the student reads aloud and along with the tape. The student continues to read along with the tape until he or she is able to read the text independently without the support of the tape.

The fourth instructional strategy recommended by the National Reading Panel (2000) was *partner reading*. Employing this strategy involves pairing students to read aloud to one another. Using this strategy, teachers can pair a stronger reader with a less fluent reader or similarly leveled readers with each other. When a stronger reader is partnered with a less fluent reader, the stronger reader may read first in order to provide a model for the less capable reader. When students with similar reading needs are paired, turn taking or choral reading can be employed.

Readers' theater is the final recommended instructional strategy. According to the National Reading Panel (2000), readers' theater provides students with the opportunity to rehearse and perform a play. This method of repeated readings offers students a reason to reread text and practice fluent, expressive reading within an appealing format. The National Reading Panel (2000) found that these five instructional strategies have a significant impact on readers' word recognition, fluency, and comprehension skills. In addition, these strategies apply to students across a range of grade levels, including skilled readers and those who are experiencing reading difficulties. The effectiveness of repeated readings and components that contributed to success among readers has been the subject of additional research since the findings of the National Reading Panel were published.

ADDITIONAL RESEARCH ON REPEATED READINGS

In 2004, Therrien conducted a meta-analysis to determine the most effective components of repeated reading interventions and their impact on the development of reading fluency and comprehension. In reporting the results of this meta-analysis, Therrien divided the studies into two distinct groups: *transfer* and *non-transfer* studies. **Transfer studies** were described as those that measured the ability of participants to generalize or transfer the gains achieved on fluently reading and comprehending one passage to the ability to fluently read and comprehend a new or novel passage. **Nontransfer studies** were those that measured participants' ability to fluently read or comprehend a passage after repeated exposures to the same passage were provided. Results of the meta-analysis indicated that repeated reading interventions improved students' fluency and comprehension. Furthermore, the conclusions drawn from this meta-analysis indicated that both students with and without disabilities benefited from repeated reading interventions.

A component analysis revealed that adult implemented interventions, corrective feedback on word errors, and the use of predetermined performance criteria were instructional factors that were most often associated with success in the transfer studies. Interventions that included a comprehension component, modeling, and charting progress also yielded some positive effects. Several components in the nontransfer studies produced positive effects as well. Providing students with a cue as to the focus (speed, fluency, or comprehension) of the reading was one component that was associated with improved fluency. Contrary to the results of the transfer studies, the absence of corrective feedback resulted in a greater effect than providing the feedback. Finally, results of the nontransfer studies indicated that students should be provided three to four opportunities to reread a passage (Therrien, 2004). In general, the summative conclusion of Therrien's meta-analysis indicated that adult implemented instruction, rereading a passage three to four times, corrective feedback, and establishing performance criteria appeared to have the greatest influence on improved fluency.

RESEARCH ON FLUENCY INSTRUCTION FOR STUDENTS WHO ARE DEAF OR HARD OF HEARING

As discussed in Chapter 4, two meta-analytic reviews exploring research conducted in the field of reading and deafness have recently been completed: Schirmer and McGough (2005) and Luckner, Sebald, Cooney, Young, and Goodwin Muir (2005/2006). These reviews provide insights into reading instructional practices currently being utilized with students who are deaf or hard of hearing. In their review, Schirmer and McGough identified two studies that they characterized to be related to reading fluency. The first study explored the time devoted to reading for 45 children, ages 5 to 10, in 10 different classrooms (Limbrick, McNaughton, & Clay, 1992). These researchers investigated the amount of time spent engaged in reading (e.g., reading independently, with a peer or teacher) and other reading-related tasks (e.g., answering questions, summarizing a passage, etc.). In addition, six case studies were completed that compared three students with high levels of engagement (i.e., amount of time spent in reading) to three with low levels. The conclusion drawn was that there was a correlation between level of engagement and level of reading achievement.

The second study identified by Schirmer and McGough (2005) was conducted by Kelly in 1995. The purpose of this study was to explore the differences between skilled and average readers' ability to read passages about both familiar and unfamiliar topics from a moving window text display. The participants of this study were nine readers, ages 16–19, who were considered average readers, and nine skilled readers, ages 15–18. Results indicated that both groups read familiar topics more readily than unfamiliar topics, but the skilled readers who were deaf or hard of hearing outperformed the average readers in terms of reading rate. In addition, observational information indicated that the average readers displayed uneven processing rhythms when compared to the skilled readers. Although these two studies were associated with reading fluency in the meta-analytic review, neither employed repeated readings nor the strategies recommended by the National Reading Panel (2000).

In their review, Luckner et al. (2005/2006) identified one study that explored the effects of employing reading fluency instruction with students who are deaf or hard of hearing. This study, conducted by Ensor and Koller (1997), investigated the effects of two different methods of repeated reading instruction with students in a residential school for the deaf. The 42 student participants were matched on factors such as reading ability, age, degree of hearing loss, and cognitive ability and randomly assigned to either the treatment or comparison group.

Students in the treatment group were asked to practice reading a passage at their instructional level three times. Each practice session lasted 15 minutes. Comparison students followed the same procedure, but they were asked to practice reading passages other than the target passage during sessions. Five sessions using five different passages were completed as part of this study. Essentially, the treatment group was engaged in a non-transfer condition while comparison students participated in a transfer condition as described by Therrien (2004) earlier in this chapter.

Results of this inquiry indicated that treatment students demonstrated significant improvements from pretest to posttest measures of rate and accuracy of reading. The performance of participants in the comparison group indicated minimal improvement. The authors of this study suggest that additional research be conducted in this area and that "[d]eaf educators, in general, should become more familiar with 'mainstream' techniques that have general acceptance in remedial and special education. Many, with only minor modifications, may assist their students in improving reading achievement" (Ensor & Koller, 1997, p. 69). As the authors of this book, we strongly agree with this statement and believe that this is the purpose of the current text: to inform deaf educators of effective, "mainstream" reading instructional practices supported by theory and research and provide suggestions for modifying them to meet the needs of students who are deaf or hard of hearing.

GUIDELINES FOR IMPLEMENTING FLUENCY INSTRUCTION

In order to choose appropriate passages for fluency instruction, the National Reading Panel (2000) recommended using text at the student's **independent** or **instructional reading level.** Text that can be read with 90% to 95% accuracy would be appropriate for fluency instruction. In addition, it is suggested that the text used for intervention should be relatively short. Passages that are 100 to 200 words in length are typically appropriate for instructional purposes. Finally, a variety of passage types, including fiction and nonfiction selections, is advised. Once an appropriate passage has been selected, fluency instruction can be implemented.

Using grade-leveled passages is an excellent way of providing repeated reading practice for students. Utilizing these selections allows teachers to increase the passage difficulty level over time. In addition to the list of teacher resources and Web sites provided at the end of this chapter, teachers can also create selections using passages from textbooks, novels, magazines, or newspaper articles. To determine the passage readability of the above selections, teachers can quickly determine a reading level using the **Flesch-Kincaid readability statistic** feature available through the Microsoft Word program.

The Flesch-Kincaid readability statistic uses the number of words per sentence and number of syllables per word to calculate grade-level readability for a given passage. The grade level displayed provides the writer of the document with a value that indicates the minimum education level (i.e., an estimate) required for the reader to be able to understand the document. The lower the score on a scale of 0–12, the easier it is to understand the document. To use this feature in Microsoft Word, re-create the text in a Word document. Under "Tools," choose "Options" and click on "Spelling and Grammar." In the grammar section, be sure that the box for "Show Readability Statistics" is checked. Once you have completed typing your text, under "Tools" choose "Spelling and Grammar" to display the readability statistics.

A caution in interpreting and using the readability statistic is offered. Although the readability statistic is reported in grade-equivalent terms (e.g., 4.3 indicating fourth grade, third month), the ability for a student to read these informal passages should not be used as a sole source in determining a student's reading level. However, the Flesch-Kincaid readability statistic is a useful tool for comparing passages to one another. This readability statistic is easy to use and allows teachers to provide students with passages of increasing difficulty for graduated fluency instruction.

To begin a fluency intervention, a teacher should first determine whether or not the student requires instruction by establishing a baseline score for the student. Establishing a baseline involves having the student orally read a select passage and then calculate the student's level of accuracy using either correct words per minute [CWPM = (number of words read ÷ number of seconds read) × 60], number of errors per minute [EPM = (number of errors ÷ time in seconds) × 60] or percentage of words read accurately per minute [WRA = (number of correct words ÷ total words read) × 60]. It is important to note that the evaluation of the above may vary. Errors are often defined as word substitutions, additions, omissions, and mispronunciations. In some cases, teachers consider self-corrections to be errors.

Goodman (1969) preferred the term *miscue* rather than *mistake* or *error*. The underlying premise of the miscue analysis is that the miscues students produce are neither accidental nor random but indicate the students' language and personal experiences. Once a student has completed the passage reading, each miscue is analyzed to determine if it was related to the context (either proceeding or following), whether it preserved the essential meaning, and whether or not the student corrected the miscue. This method allows the rater to determine both the quantity and quality (i.e., type) of miscues that occurred during passage reading.

How errors or miscues are defined by teachers using informal assessments might not be so important; however, it is important that this information be clearly communicated to students and those who are interpreting the results. In addition, guidelines for judging CWPM, EPM, or WRA should be consistently applied. It is important to note that when using norm-referenced measures of reading fluency, teachers must following the procedures outlined by the authors of the assessment or the results will be considered invalid.

Although the National Reading Panel (2000) did not provide guidelines for performance criteria for reading fluency, Hasbrouck and Tindal (1992, 2006) published norms for reading fluency for students with typical hearing in grades 1–8. The current norms were established by analyzing data collected from schools and districts in 23 states from 2000–2004. These detailed norms include percentiles from the 10th through 90th level for students at three points during the school year: fall, winter, and spring. Using this information, teachers can determine how students compare to the normative sample and whether or not fluency instruction is warranted. Table 5-1 provides the correct words per minute by grade and percentile level. The 50th percentile is considered average for each grade level.

TABLE 5-1   Fluency Norms

| Grade | Percentile | Correct Words per Minute | | |
		Fall	Winter	Spring
1	90	n/a	81	111
	75	n/a	47	82
	50	*n/a*	23	53
	25	n/a	12	28
	10	n/a	6	15
2	90	106	125	142
	75	79	100	117
	50	*51*	72	89
	25	25	42	61
	10	11	18	31

TABLE 5-1 Fluency Norms (Cont'd)

Grade	Percentile	Correct Words per Minute		
		Fall	Winter	Spring
3	90	128	146	162
	75	99	120	137
	50	*71*	*92*	*107*
	25	44	62	78
	10	21	36	48
4	90	145	166	180
	75	119	139	152
	50	*94*	*112*	*123*
	25	68	87	98
	10	45	61	72
5	90	166	182	194
	75	139	156	168
	50	*110*	*127*	*139*
	25	85	99	109
	10	61	74	83
6	90	177	195	204
	75	153	167	177
	50	*127*	*140*	*150*
	25	98	111	122
	10	68	82	93
7	90	180	192	202
	75	156	165	177
	50	*128*	*136*	*150*
	25	102	109	123
	10	79	88	98
8	90	185	199	199
	75	161	173	177
	50	*133*	*146*	*151*
	25	106	115	124
	10	77	84	97

Source: Adapted from Hasbrouck and Tindal (2006)

TABLE 5-2   Assessments of Fluency

Name of Assessment	Copyright	Publisher	Web Site
AIMSweb	2007	Harcourt	http://aimsweb.com
Dynamic Indicators of Basic Early Literacy Skills, 6th edition (DIBELS-6)	2007	University of Oregon	http://dibels.uoregon.edu/
Gray Oral Reading Test, 4th edition (GORT-4)	2001	Pearson Assessments	http://ags.pearsonassessments.com
Fluency: Strategies and Assessments (2nd edition)	2005	Kendall/Hunt	http://www.kendallhunt.com
Reading Fluency Benchmark Assessor	2007	Read Naturally	http://www.readnaturally.com
Test of Silent Word Reading Fluency (TOSWRF)	2004	ProEd	http://www.proedinc.com
Texas Primary Reading Inventory (TPRI)	2006	Texas Education Agency University of Texas System	http://www.tpri.org

Once a student's baseline is compared to the norms provided, the need for fluency instruction can be determined. If it is decided that the student would benefit from fluency instruction, the teacher can employ one of the five research-based instructional strategies outlined by the National Reading Panel (2000) and consider integrating the components that were consistently associated with successful repeated reading interventions (Therrien, 2004).

ASSESSMENTS OF FLUENCY

Informal assessments of reading fluency usually involve the use of curriculum-based measures. Monitoring students' CWPM on grade-leveled passages would be considered a curriculum-based measure. Benchmark assessments are now commonly used to compare students' oral reading fluency measures to established norms or benchmarks. As with phonemic awareness and phonics assessments included in Chapter 4, a search of the Southwest Educational Development Laboratory [SEDL] (2007) online database of reading

assessments for students in kindergarten to second grade was conducted. This search yielded only two results, but additional assessments were drawn from alternative sources (e.g., Hasbrouck & Tindal, 2006). The names of the assessments, copyright, publisher, and Web site for each assessment is summarized in Table 5-2. As discussed in Chapter 4, it is important for test administrators to review each subtest carefully to determine the effects of various administrative procedures to ensure that valid results are obtained, particularly for students who are deaf or hard of hearing.

QUESTIONS SURROUNDING IMPLEMENTING READING FLUENCY INTERVENTIONS WITH STUDENTS WHO ARE DEAF OR HARD OF HEARING

Several questions arise when considering implementing fluency instruction for students who are deaf or hard of hearing. Considering the hierarchical nature of reading skill development delineated by Chall (1996), the first question that comes to mind is: Have students who are deaf or hard of hearing achieved adequate automaticity with word recognition skills to warrant attention to fluency instruction? As described in Chapter 2 of this text, Chall indicated that the progression through the stages of reading development depends on the acquisition and mastery of skills at the previous stage. Chall labeled her third stage in the reading development process *confirmation and fluency*. The prerequisite skills for this stage include direct instruction in letter–sound relationships or phonics. As discussed in Chapter 4, studies evaluating this type of instruction with students who are deaf or hard of hearing are just beginning to emerge in the literature (see Trezek & Malmgren, 2005; Trezek & Wang, 2006; Trezek, Wang, Woods, Gampp & Paul, 2007). Automaticity in identifying letter–sound relationships is a precursor to automatic word recognition that in turn leads to sentence-level fluency and finally the ability to fluently read connected text. Therefore, the first step to improving reading fluency for students who are deaf or hard of hearing may involve developing automaticity at the sound, word, and sentence levels.

For those students who have established adequate word-identification skills and who can read words in connected text, the second question that arises is: Do fluency norms that have been established for hearing readers apply to students who are deaf or hard of hearing? Even though deaf or hard of hearing students were not part of the norming sample, there is a practical response: The answer to this question may vary, depending on the student. Consider the student who utilizes speech production when reading and therefore is capable of orally reading passages in a manner similar to a hearing peer. In this case, the teacher must determine whether or not the student's attention to proper articulation plays a role in his oral reading fluency. Attention to correct articulation may in fact affect the rate of oral reading for the student, so not allowing him to meet the correct word per minute criterion established for his particular grade level.

In this situation, we suggest that teachers establish a percentage over the student's own baseline as a goal when implementing fluency instruction. For example, suppose that the student is reading at a rate of 50 words per minute. In fluency exercises, the goal may be to have the student engage in repeated reading tasks until he can read at a rate 40% above his baseline. This rate of increase has been recommended by several authors as a percentage of increase that will generalize to increased rates when presented with a new or novel passage (e.g., Carnine, Silbert, Kame'enui & Tarver, 2004). Given the example of the student reading 50 words per minute, the teacher would set a target rate at 70 words per minute $(50 + [40\%$ of $50 = 20] = 70)$. If a student were reading at a rate of 90 words per minute, then the target rate would be 126 per minute $(90 + [40\%$ of $90 = 36] = 126)$. Using this method of goal setting, the rate of reading and goal for improvement are based on the student's own baseline level.

The third question that surfaces is: How do we adapt reading fluency instruction for students who use a form of sign language as their main mode of communication? The aforementioned method of goal setting 40% above the student's baseline rate can certainly be used with students who utilize sign language to read passages. Additional factors to consider when employing reading fluency interventions with students who use either an English sign system (e.g., Signed English, Signing Exact English) or American Sign Language (ASL) were summarized by Easterbrooks and Huston (2008). These authors also developed a definition of signed fluency and rubric for evaluating the presence of absence of skills among readers who are deaf or hard of hearing. The process they used to develop the rubric and results of applying the rubric to evaluate the signed reading fluency of middle school students who are deaf or hard of hearing is described in the following section.

Signed Reading Fluency Rubric for Deaf Children

In developing the definition of signed reading fluency and a rubric for determining students' fluency levels, characteristics associated with both proficiency in signed communication and literacy were used. Signed stories presented by skilled readers who were deaf and utilized ASL were viewed to determine important aspects of fluent, signed presentations. According to the authors (Easterbrooks & Huston, 2008), the evaluation of signed reading fluency involves assessing skills in three general categories: *accuracy, fluency envelope,* and *visual grammar. Accuracy* was defined as the "ability of the signer to render the concepts in English print text into a signed format that has equivalent conceptual meaning" (Easterbrooks & Huston, 2008, p. 42). The authors suggest that teachers use miscue analysis or other informal or formal assessments to measure the accuracy of student reading. The *fluency envelope* is described as the overall appearance of the signed message and contains elements that convey the mood and intent and essentially display the pragmatic aspects of the text. Factors to consider include speed of signing, facial expressions, body movements, sign movement, and the use of sign space and

finger spelling. The category *visual grammar* is used to assess students' ability to express the syntactic aspects of literacy and includes components such as use of space, role taking, eye gaze, negation (through head shaking or body language), directionality of sign, sign classifiers, and pronominalization (using indexing rather than English signs for *he, she, them,* etc.).

Using the analysis discussed above, Easterbrooks and Huston (2008) developed a rubric to assess students' skills in the areas of fluency envelope and visual grammar. To utilize the developed rubric, teachers videotape students reading a narrative text at their independent reading level. The rater can then watch the video tape and judge the students' signed representation of text using a 0–4 rating:

0—not observed

1—emerging

2—beginning

3—developing

4—mature or fluent

Descriptors of skills and level of performance also accompany each numerical rating. The ratings for both the fluency envelope and visual grammar categories are then translated into an overall signed reading fluency score indicating poor, emerging, beginning, developing, or mature signed reading fluency. After the rubric was developed, three trained evaluators assessed seven middle school students' signed reading fluency in order to conduct interrater reliability measures on the rubric that was developed. These evaluations resulted in ratings from 0.975 to 1.00, indicating that the developed rubric yielded highly reliable results.

The rubric was then used to assess the signed reading fluency of 29 middle school students who were deaf or hard of hearing attending a day school for the deaf in a large metropolitan city. Participants were assessed over the course of an academic year using both the developed Signed Reading Fluency Rubric for Deaf Children and the Word and Passage Comprehension subtests of the Woodcock Reading Mastery Test–Revised (WRMT-R). In general, results of the WRMT-R assessments indicated that the participants had reading comprehension scores that were lower than their same-aged hearing peers (Easterbrooks & Huston, 2008).

Results of this inquiry indicated that there was a positive correlation between scores on the Signed Reading Fluency Rubric for Deaf Children and scores on the standardized measures of word and reading comprehension. The strongest relationships were noted between ratings of the fluency envelope and passage comprehension and total fluency and passage comprehension. In other words, higher signed reading fluency scores were associated with higher scores on measures of reading comprehension (Easterbrooks & Huston, 2008). These results mirror the findings obtained with hearing readers, indicating that there is a relationship between reading fluency and comprehension. As the authors of this text, we suggest that future research investigations of fluency employ the Signed Reading Fluency Rubric for Deaf Children to evaluate the effects of repeated reading interventions conducted with signing students who are deaf or hard of hearing.

INSTRUCTIONAL GOALS AND OBJECTIVES

As discussed in Chapter 4, teachers are required to include instructional goals and objectives to meet the needs outlined in students' Individualized Education Programs. In the present level of performance, the teacher describes the student's need in a particular area and includes relevant information collected via assessment. The annual goal describes, in measurable terms, what can reasonably be accomplished given a year of instruction. The short-term objectives or benchmarks are then crafted to divide the annual goal into discrete instructional components. A sample annual goal along with short-term objectives to address a need in the area of reading fluency is included in Table 5-3. This sample instructional goal is written to address Brianna's fluency needs, the student who is the subject of Case Study B. For further information regarding Brianna, please refer to the information provided in the case study section of the text.

FLUENCY INSTRUCTION INCLUDED IN CORE READING CURRICULA

As discussed in Chapter 4, the American Federation of Teachers has recommended the use of *A Consumer's Guide to Evaluating a Core Reading Program, Grades K–3: A Critical Elements Analysis* (Simmons & Kame'enui, 2003) to evaluate the components of commercially available curricula for reading instruction for kindergarten through third-grade students. According to the guidelines in the consumer guide, fluency instruction was considered an essential skill that should be included in reading curriculum for first- through third-grade students. For purposes of this chapter on fluency instruction, the evaluation of the nine different reading programs conducted by the Oregon Reading First Center (2004) was

---

TABLE 5-3 Annual Goal and Short-Term Objectives for Fluency

Area of Need: Reading Fluency

Present Level of Performance:
On the fall benchmark assessment of the Dynamic Indicators of Basic Early Literacy Skills (DIBELS), Brianna's median score of the three passage readings was 68 correct words per minute. According to the normative data of the DIBELS assessment, fourth graders reading less than 71 correct words per minute (CWPM) are considered at risk in the area of reading fluency. Although Brianna's reading is relatively accurate, she reads word by word and therefore her rate of reading is slow. An informal assessment of reading fluency supports the results obtained on the DIBELS. When given a fourth-grade-leveled passage, Brianna was able to correctly read 65 words per minute. According the norms provided by Hasbrouck and Tindal (2006), this rate falls below the 25th percentile. In addition to her difficulties in the area of rate, Brianna's expression and phrasing during oral reading tasks warrants attention.

Goal:
Given opportunities to engage in repeated reading exercises, Brianna will increase her reading fluency to the 50th percentile (123 CWPM) by the end of the spring quarter.

How will progress toward this goal be measured?
Graded reading passage, teacher observations, progress log sheets, parent and student reports

Short-term objectives or benchmarks including criteria for evaluation

- Given a grade leveled passage, Brianna will engage in repeated readings until she is able to achieve a 40% over baseline gain before practicing a new passage.

- Following each oral passage reading, Brianna will request feedback regarding both her rate and accuracy.

- Brianna will chart her fluency progress on a log sheet at the end of each repeated reading session.

- Given an adult model of fluent and expressive reading, Brianna will reread the modeled passage at least two times during the week to practice expression and proper phrasing.

- Brianna will practice reading selected passages with an adult at home at least two times per week.

Progress Toward Annual Goal

Date	Progress*	Comments:

*Minimal (M): anticipate that the goal will not be met by the end of the quarter
Proficient (P): anticipate that the goal will be met by the end of the quarter
Advanced (A): anticipate that the goal will be exceeded by the end of the quarter

---

reviewed. The evaluation included the following nine curricula: *Hartcourt, Houghton Mifflin, Macmillian/McGraw-Hill, Open Court, Reading Mastery, Rigby Literacy, Scott Foresman, Success for All,* and *Wright Group.*

Curricula with the highest percentage ratings in the high-priority category for fluency instruction at the first-grade level include *Success for All* (88%), *Harcourt* (83%), *Reading Mastery* (83%), and *Houghton Mifflin* and *Scott Foresman* (75%). At the second-grade level, the top-rated programs for fluency instruction include *Reading Mastery* (100%), *Houghton Mifflin* (92%), *Open Court* (83%), and *Harcourt* and *Scott Foresman* (75%). Finally, the curricula that included the strongest fluency instruction for third-grade readers are *Open Court* (92%), *Reading Mastery* (83%), *Harcourt* and *Houghton Mifflin* (67%), and *Macmillian/McGraw-Hill* (58%).

As with phonemic awareness and phonics instruction, we encourage readers to explore the curricula above or use the Consumer's Guide (Simmons & Kame'enui, 2003) or both to evaluate curricula not included in this review in order to identify effective, comprehensive, beginning reading curriculums to implement with students who are deaf or hard of hearing. In addition to published reading curricula, there are many print and online resources available to provide teachers with ideas for teaching and reinforcing reading fluency. A list of these teacher resources is included at the end of this chapter. In addition, teacher-created materials may also be utilized to address reading fluency instruction. A description of several activities is provided in the following section.

FLUENCY INSTRUCTIONAL ACTIVITIES

The National Reading Panel (2000) defines reading fluency as the ability to read a passage accurately, quickly, and with proper expression. As discussed earlier in this chapter, some students may need to develop automaticity with sound identification and word reading as well as fluency with sentence reading before instructional activities can focus on the development of reading fluency at the passage level. Therefore, the following activities address the development of fluency at the sound, word, sentence, and passage levels.

Sound and Word-Level Fluency

- *Clear the Table:* To prepare for this activity, the teacher would write sounds or words that require repetition to achieve automaticity on small paper plates. The plates can then be placed upside down on a table. Students *clear the table* by reading the sounds or words on the plates, but they can only remove the plate from the table if the sound or word is read correctly. Given a one-minute time limit, students can record their scores and document their progress over time. In addition, students can challenge each other to a race.

- *Sound or Word Flash:* This activity begins with the teacher reviewing word flash cards containing targeted sounds or words for practice. Once the students are comfortable with the sounds or words, the teacher divides the students into groups of three. One student plays the role of game show host, and the other two act as contestants. To play the game, the host places a flash card face up on the table. Whichever contestant can tap the table first to indicate that he knows the sound or word is given the opportunity to read the sound or word. If he is correct, the card is earned. The contestant with the most cards at the end of a two-minute period wins that round, and students rotate roles and begin another round of *Sound* or *Word Flash*.

- *Word Walk:* To prepare this activity, the teacher can write sounds or words that require practice on footprint-shaped pieces of paper and tape them to the floor around the classroom. Using a timer, a student will begin the footprint path saying the correct sound or word before proceeding to the next footprint. The goal is to see how quickly he can reach the end of the path, and he can be challenged to beat his previous time. As with the *Clear the Table* activity, students can record their progress over time. Additional practice on these sounds and/or words can be provided throughout the school day. Each time the student passes over a footprint during the day, they must say the correct sound or word.

Sentence-Level Fluency

- *Perform the Poem:* Poetry is an excellent medium for practicing sentence fluency because reading a poem requires a student to read words in phrases rather than word by word. This activity can begin by having the teacher provide a model of poem reading. This will also ensure that the students know all the words contained in the poem. Once the poem has been read by the teacher, she can lead the group through several choral readings. Students can also be divided into groups or partners and take turns reciting the poem. Once adequate practice has occurred, a student can perform the poem for his class.

- *Marks Make a Difference:* The development of prosody or expressive reading can begin with sentence-level fluency practice. Students can practice reciting simple sentences that use various punctuations to focus on the intonation required when a different mark is employed. For example, "Dogs bark. Dogs bark? Dogs bark!" Simple sentences can also be used to practice emphasizing various words in the sentence such as "*We* are happy. We *are* happy. We are *happy.*" The class can then discuss how intonation affects the way the message is perceived.

- *Sentence Dash:* This activity begins by preparing a list of short phrases and displaying them on a piece of paper in three columns; beginnings, middles, and endings (see Table 5-4). The goal of the activity is to see how many sentences the student can combine and accurately read in one minute. The paper can also be cut into

TABLE 5-4 Sentence Dash

Beginnings	Middles	Endings
The little boy	road a bike	to the store.
Dad	ran from the house	to catch a bus.
Mom	was in a hurry	to get to work.
My teacher	wanted	to eat lunch.
The children	waited	in the line.

strips for students to be able to physically manipulate the sentences. The number and complexity of beginnings, middles, and endings that the teacher provides varies depending on the students' ages and skill levels.

Passage-Level Fluency

- *Action!:* Readers' theater is an excellent way to promote reading fluency at the passage level. Any short story or chapter in a book can easily be adapted for this activity. In addition to the practice students receive with fluency, this activity is a wonderful way to expose students to a variety of genres of literature (e.g., folk tales, mythology) as well as reinforce the use of quotation marks and dialogue.

- *Solve a Mystery:* To prepare for this activity, the teacher presents a short mystery to students in which each paragraph is printed on a separate piece of paper. Dividing the class into teams, each member of the group must read his section of the mystery to the group. Once the first reading is completed, the students must place the pieces of the mystery in the correct order. Once this is achieved, students will reread the mystery, each one taking a turn and reading his part. In addition to fluency, this activity emphasizes sequencing and comprehension. A nice resource of mystery stories created by children and for children is available online at http://kids.mysterynet.com/.

- *Recite a Rap:* After they read a story selection or chapter in a book, have students work in groups to create a rap, poem, or song that summarizes the selection read. After they complete their writing, students can reread and practice their creation before they recite their rap for the class. This activity focuses not only on fluency but also on writing, comprehension, and rhyming if desired.

CONCLUSION

This chapter focused on the importance of fluency instruction for children and adolescents who are deaf or hard of hearing. The discussion was guided by the recommendations of the National Reading Panel (2000), a meta-analysis that summarized repeated reading interventions (Therrien, 2004), as well as by a synthesis of the available research on individuals who are deaf or hard of hearing. When implementing fluency instruction for students who are deaf or hard of hearing, three questions should be considered: (1) Have students who are deaf or hard of hearing achieved adequate automaticity with word-recognition skills to warrant attention to fluency instruction? (2) Do fluency norms that have been established for hearing readers apply to students who are deaf or hard of hearing? (3) How do we adapt reading fluency instruction for students who use a form of sign language as their main mode of communication? Answers to these questions were discussed in detail in this chapter.

CHAPTER SUMMARY

- Fluency is the ability to read a text accurately and quickly with proper expression. The findings of the National Reading Panel (2000) conclude that guided, repeated oral reading proves more promising than independent silent reading. Five of the recommended instructional strategies for promoting fluent reading are student–adult, choral, tape-assisted, and partner reading as well as readers' theater.

- Therrien's (2004) meta-analysis of effective components of repeated reading interventions divided studies into two distinct groups: *transfer* and *nontransfer studies.* Transfer studies were those that measured the ability of participants to generalize or transfer the gains achieved on fluently reading or comprehending one new or novel passage. Nontransfer studies were those that measured participants' ability to fluently read or comprehend a repeated passage. Results of Therrien's (2004) meta-analysis indicated that repeated reading interventions improved students' fluency and comprehension and that both students with and without disabilities benefited from repeated reading interventions.

- Schirmer and McGough's (2005) meta-analytic review on reading research of students who are deaf or hard of hearing identified two studies associated with reading fluency, but neither employed repeated readings or the strategies recommended by the National Reading Panel (2000).

- Three questions are investigated regarding implementing fluency instruction for students who are deaf or hard of hearing: (1) Have students who are deaf or hard of hearing achieved adequate automaticity with word-recognition skills to warrant attention to fluency instruction? (2) Do fluency norms that have been established for hearing readers apply to students who are deaf or hard of hearing? (3) How do we adapt reading fluency instruction for students who use a form of sign language as their main mode of communication?

- Easterbrooks and Huston (2008) suggested that the evaluation of signed reading

fluency involved assessing skills in three general categories: *accuracy*, *fluency envelope*, and *visual grammar*. The results of the signed reading fluency study for students who are deaf or hard of hearing mirrored the findings obtained with hearing readers, indicating that there is a relationship between reading fluency and comprehension.

REVIEW QUESTIONS

1. What are the key components of fluency defined by National Reading Panel (2000)?

2. According to National Reading Panel (2000), comparing guided, repeated oral reading and independent silent reading, which practice yields the best result in promoting fluent reading? What are the five recommended instructional strategies for promoting fluent reading?

3. How can it be determined whether or not a student requires fluency instruction?

4. When implementing fluency instruction for students who are deaf or hard of hearing, what are some questions that should be asked?

5. According to Easterbrooks and Huston (2008), how can the signed reading fluency of students who are deaf or hard of hearing be evaluated?

REFLECTIVE QUESTIONS

1. Using the examples provided in this chapter as your guide, create two instructional activities to promote fluent reading for students who are deaf of hard of hearing.

2. How do we adapt the five recommended instructional strategies identified by

National Reading Panel (2000) in promoting fluent reading for students who use a form of sign language as their main mode of communication?

APPLICATION EXERCISES

1. Using the annual goal and objective presented in this chapter, write a week-long fluency lesson plan to address one of

the short-term objectives written for Brianna.

2. Write a present level of performance, an annual goal, and at least three short-term objectives to address the reading fluency needs of Danielle, the subject of Case Study D.

SUGGESTED READINGS AND RESOURCES

Readings

Adams, G., & Brown, S. (2007). *The six-minute solution: A reading fluency program (primary level).* Longmont, CO: Sopris West.

Adams, G., & Brown, S. (2007). *The six-minute solution: A reading fluency program (intermediate level).* Longmont, CO: Sopris West.

Barchers, S. I. (1997). *Fifty fabulous fables. Beginning readers theatre.* Portsmouth, NH: Teachers Idea Press.

Blevins, W. (2001). *Building fluency: Lessons and strategies for reading success.* New York: Scholastic Professional Books.

Fredericks, A. D. (1997). *Tadpole tales and other totally terrific treats for readers theatre.* Westport, CT: Greenwood Publishing Group.

Hiskes, D. G. (2007). *Reading pathways: Simple exercises to improve reading fluency.* San Francisco: Jossey-Bass.

Rasinski, T. V. (2003). *The fluent reading: Oral reading strategies for building word recognition, fluency and comprehension.* New York: Scholastic Professional Books.

Rasinski, T. V., Blachowicz, C., & Lems, K. (2006). *Fluency instruction: Research-based best practices.* New York: Guilford Press.

Resources

Curriculum-Based Measurement Warehouse http://www.interventioncentral.org/htmdocs/interventions/cbmwarehouse.php

Intervention Central: Custom Reading Probes http://www.interventioncentral.org/htmdocs/tools/okapi/okapi.php

Joe Witt Reading Center http://www.joewitt.org/reading/

Reading a-z.com: The Online Reading Program http://www.readinga-z.com

University of Southern Maine—College of Education and Human Development http://www.usm.maine.edu/cehd/assessment-center/C-BM.htm

REFERENCES

Armbruster, B. B., Lehr, F., & Osborn, J. (2001). *Put reading first: The research building blocks for teaching children to read kindergarten through grade three.* Jessup, MD: National Institute for Literacy.

Carnine, D. W., Silbert, J., Kame'enui, E. J., & Tarver, S. G. (2004). *Direct instruction reading.* (4th ed.). Upper Saddle River, NJ: Pearson Education.

Chall, J. S. (1996). *Stages of reading development.* (2nd ed.). New York: McGraw-Hill.

Ensor, A. D., & Koller, J. R. (1997). The effects of the method of repeated readings on reading rate and word recognition accuracy of deaf adolescents. *Journal of Deaf Studies and Deaf Education*, 2, 61–70.

Easterbrooks, S. R. & Huston, S. G. (2008). The signed reading fluency of students who are deaf/hard of hearing. *Journal of Deaf Studies and Deaf Education*. 13 (1), 37–54.

Goodman, K. (1969). Analysis of oral reading miscues: Applied psycholinguistics. In F. Gollasch (Ed.) *Language and literacy: The selected writings of Kenneth Goodman* (pp. 123–134). Vol. I. Boston: Routledge & Kegan Paul.

Hasbrouck, J. E., & Tindal, G. (1992). Curriculum-based oral reading fluency norms for students in grades 2–5. *Teaching Exceptional Children*, 24 (3), p. 41–44.

Hasbrouck, J., & Tindal, G. A. (2006). Oral reading fluency norms: A valuable assessment tool for reading teachers. *International Reading Association*, 59 (7), 636–644.

Kelly, L. P. (1995). Processing of bottom-up and top-down information by skilled and average deaf readers and implications for whole language instruction. *Exceptional Children*, 61, 318–334.

Limbrick, E. A., McNaughton, S., & Clay, M. M. (1992). Time engaged in reading: A critical factor in reading achievement. *American Annals of the Deaf*, 137, 309–314.

Luckner, J. L., Sebald, A. N., Cooney, J., Young, J., & Goodwin Muir, S. (2005/2006). An examination of the evidence-based literacy research in deaf education. *American Annals of the Deaf*, 150 (5), 443–456.

National Reading Panel (2000). *Report of the National Reading Panel: Teaching children to read — An evidence-based assessment of the scientific research literature on reading and its implications for reading instruction*. Jessup, MD: National Institute for Literacy at EDPubs.

Oregon Reading First Center. (2004). *Review of Comprehensive Reading Programs*. Retrieved October 21, 2007, from http:// reading.uoregon.edu/curricula/intro_ summ_review_3-04.pdf.

Schirmer, B. R., & McGough, S. M. (2005). Teaching reading to children who are deaf: Do the conclusions of the National Reading Panel apply? *Review of Educational Research*, 75 (1), 83–117.

Simmons, D. C., & Kame'enui, E. J. (2003). *A consumer's guide to evaluating a core reading program, grades K-3: A critical elements analysis*. Retrieved October 21, 2007, from http://teacher.scholastic.com/ products/fundingconnection/pdf/Kameenui_GR_Blue.pdf

Snow, C. E., Burns, S. M., & Griffin, P. (Eds.). (1998). *Preventing reading difficulties in young children*. Washington, DC: National Academy Press.

Southwest Educational Development Laboratory (2007). *Reading assessment database*. Retrieved March 3, 2007 from http:// www.sedl.org/reading/rad/database.html.

Therrien, W. (2004). Fluency and comprehension gains as a result of repeated reading: A meta-analysis. *Remedial and Special Education*, 25, 252–261.

Trezek, B. J., & Malmgren, K. W. (2005). The efficacy of utilizing a phonics treatment package with middle school deaf and hard-of-hearing students.*Journal of Deaf Studies and Deaf Education*, 3, 257–271.

Trezek, B. J., & Wang, Y. (2006). Implications of utilizing a phonics-based reading curriculum with children who are deaf or hard of hearing.*Journal of Deaf Studies and Deaf Education, 11* (2), 202–213.

Trezek, B. J., Wang, Y., Woods, D. G., Gampp, T. L., & Paul, P. (2007). Using Visual Phonics to supplement beginning reading instruction for students who are deaf or hard of hearing.*Journal of Deaf Studies and Deaf Education, 12* (3), 373–384.

CHAPTER 6

VOCABULARY

Much conventional wisdom about vocabulary instruction fluctuates between two poles: read a lot or make a weekly word list for a Friday quiz. Neither pole is the true north magnet for vocabulary growth with a lasting impact on reading achievement. What does work is well-planned instruction that provokes student engagement in different situations so that new words are used, feedback is given, and students make personal connections among new and known vocabulary items (Snow, Griffin, & Burns, 2005, p. 90).

CHAPTER OBJECTIVES

After completing this chapter, the reader will be able to:

- Describe the National Reading Panel's findings relative to vocabulary instruction
- Explain the research exploring the efficacy of vocabulary instruction with students who are deaf or hard of hearing
- Discuss appropriate Individualized Education Program (IEP) goals and short-term objectives for vocabulary instruction
- Create instructional activities to teach vocabulary

INTRODUCTION

*T*he purpose of reading is comprehension. Comprehension at the word level is considered vocabulary. As beginning readers, children make sense of the words they see in print by using the words they have heard or said. Vocabulary plays a critical role in comprehension because readers need to understand what most of the words mean to gain meaning from a text. Meanwhile, to be successful in the classrooms, children must understand the vocabulary used by the teacher in presenting rules, directions, and demonstrations. Therefore, developing adequate vocabulary skills not only is crucial to reading skills such as comprehending individual words in print or understanding the meaning of written selections, but also contributes greatly to general school success (Carnine, Silbert, Kame'enui, Tarver, & Jungjohann, 2004).

Summarizing the findings of more than 100 years of vocabulary research, Graves and Watts-Taffe (2002) concluded that (1) vocabulary knowledge is one of the best predictors of verbal ability, (2) vocabulary difficulty significantly influences the readability of text, (3) children growing up in poverty and other disadvantaged children are more likely to have substantially smaller vocabulary before entering school and are less likely to maintain an adequate vocabulary, and (4) lack of vocabulary can be a critical factor underlying the school failure of disadvantaged students. In light of the critical role vocabulary plays, what are the best ways to teach vocabulary?

In this chapter, the National Reading Panel's (2000) conclusions and suggestions for instruction in the area of vocabulary are described in greater detail. Studies exploring the efficacy of using these vocabulary instructional techniques with students who are deaf or hard of hearing are also reviewed. Guidelines for implementing vocabulary instruction with students are discussed, and an overview of several assessments of vocabulary is supplied. A sample Individualized Education Program (IEP) goal and objectives to address vocabulary needs are provided. Evaluations of selected curricula that incorporate vocabulary instruction as well as sample vocabulary instructional activities are also included. In the conclusion, major points are highlighted, and directions for future research discussed.

VOCABULARY

Vocabulary refers to the words we must know to comprehend and communicate effectively. There are four different types of vocabulary: (1) **listening vocabulary** (i.e., the words we need to know to understand what we hear), (2) **speaking vocabulary** (i.e., the words we use when we speak), (3) **reading vocabulary** (i.e., the words we need to know to understand what we read), and (4) **writing vocabulary** (i.e., the words we use in writing). Listening vocabulary and speaking vocabulary are also referred to as **oral vocabulary**—that is, the words we use in speaking or we recognize while listening (Armbruster, Lehr, & Osborn, 2001).

According to the National Reading Panel (2000), the scientific research on vocabulary instruction concludes that although some vocabulary must be taught directly, the majority of vocabulary is learned indirectly. Children's indirect vocabulary learning occurs in various contexts: engaging daily in oral language, listening to adults read to them, and reading extensively on their own. Direct vocabulary instruction for children should provide students with specific word instruction and teach word-learning strategies. In addition, teachers need to foster word consciousness in students to help them develop vocabulary. A detailed explanation of these vocabulary types of instruction is discussed in the following sections.

Indirect Vocabulary Learning

The vocabulary of a typically developing child increases approximately 3,000 new words every year or roughly 8 new words each day (Nagy & Anderson, 1984). It is generally accepted by researchers that it is impossible for children to learn such a magnitude of vocabulary through direct classroom instruction alone (Carnine, Silbert, Kame'enui, & Tarver, 2004). Thus, the meanings of most words in their vocabulary must be learned indirectly through everyday experience with oral and written language such as through conversation with adults, listening to adults read to them, and reading extensively on their own.

Beginning readers are only able to read a small portion of the words in their receptive and expressive vocabularies in print; therefore, adult–child communication in oral language is critical during the early stages. The more oral language experience children have, the more word meanings they acquire (Armbruster et al., 2001). Many students do not enter school with adequate vocabulary and sufficient oral language skills, so they are at risk of failure in reading unless they are provided with reinforced instruction in basic vocabulary and oral language. Teachers need to provide a language-enriched milieu in which students can engage in extended and productive learning with vocabulary. The importance of early oral language competence is also reinforced and emphasized in Chall's (1996) Stage 0 (see discussion in Chapter 2). Chall indicated that the development of skills at this prereading stage involves being immersed in a literate, print-rich culture and is highly dependent on interactions with adults. According to Chall, students who enter school with improvised vocabulary knowledge will require additional, possibly specialized, instruction.

Reading aloud to children is one of the most effective means of assisting vocabulary building. During such reading sessions, an adult should discuss the selection before reading, pause during reading to define unfamiliar words, and engage the child in a conversation about the book afterward. Dialogues about books not only help children learn new words and concepts, but also assist them in relating the vocabulary to their **prior knowledge** and experience (Armbruster et al., 2001).

More advanced readers can learn vocabulary indirectly through reading on their own. Research indicates that by the third grade, the amount of time children spent free reading is the major determinant of their vocabulary growth (Nagy, Anderson, & Herman, 1987). However, researchers also advise that learning word meanings from independent reading alone is not a sufficient way to build vocabulary. For example, children will only independently learn between 5 and 15 of 100 unfamiliar words they meet in reading (Nagy, Herman, & Anderson, 1985). Therefore, they must read extensively to learn a sizable amount of unfamiliar words. Furthermore, children must become fluent readers first to engage in free reading as a sufficient way of improving vocabulary (Carnine, Silbert, Kame'enui, & Tarver, 2004). These findings are also echoed in Chall's (1996) descriptions of skill development as Stages 1 and 2 (see discussion in Chapter 2). Without intact automatic word-identification skills and the ability to read connected text fluency, the transition to Stage 3 reading that allows children to use reading as a tool for learning new vocabulary and content is significantly hampered.

Direct Vocabulary Learning

For beginning readers with limited decoding skills, explicit vocabulary instruction may be most appropriate to promote vocabulary development. Even for fluent readers, explicit vocabulary instruction may be used to enhance more contextual and natural learning strategies (Carnine, Silbert, Kame'enui, & Tarver, 2004; National Reading Panel, 2000). Regardless of the skill level of the reader, the National Reading Panel recommended two instructional methods—specific word instruction and teaching word-learning strategies—to foster vocabulary development among students.

Specific Word Instruction

One direct vocabulary instructional strategy is specific word instruction (i.e., teaching individual words), which serves to deepen students' knowledge of word meanings. Given that only approximately 8 or 10 new words can be taught thoroughly per week (Armbruster et al., 2001), it is important to consider what kind of words should be taught. According to the National Reading Panel (2000), three types of words should be the focus of teaching: important words, useful words, and difficult words. *Important words* are those that are essential to

understanding the passage. *Useful words* are those that students will find handy in many contexts—for example, high-frequency words. *Difficult words* include words with multiple meanings, words with the same spelling or pronunciation, and idiomatic expressions (Armbruster et al., 2001).

Particularly, research suggests that the following practices will improve vocabulary learning and aids reading comprehension accordingly: (1) teaching specific words before reading, (2) extended instruction that promotes active engagement with vocabulary, and (3) repeated exposure to vocabulary in various contexts (Armbruster et al., 2001).

Teach Word-Learning Strategies

In addition to direct vocabulary instruction, word-learning strategies should also be emphasized so that students are able to develop effective strategies to determine the meaning of words that are new to them but not taught directly to them. Skilled readers are not readers who know every word but readers who manage effectively with words that are new to them (Carnine, Silbert, Kame'enui, & Tarver, 2004; Irvin, 1998). Word-learning strategies include using the following to determine word meanings: (1) dictionaries and other reference aids; (2) information on within-word parts—for example, *prefixes* (i.e., word parts that are "fixed" to the beginnings of words), *suffixes* (i.e., word parts that are "fixed" to the ending of words), *base words* (i.e., words from which many other words are formed), and *root words* (i.e., words from other languages that are the origin of many English words); and (3) context clues (Armbruster et al., 2001). As discussed in Chapter 2, Chall (1996) also recommended systematic word study to improve and enhance reading skills for readers in Stage 4 and beyond.

Word Consciousness

Word consciousness refers to an awareness of and interest in words, their meanings, and their power and involves both a cognitive and an affective perspective toward words. Word-conscious students know many words, know how to learn new words, enjoy words, and are eager to learn them (Stahl & Nagy, 2006). "With tens of thousands of words to learn and with most of this word learning taking place incidentally as learners are reading and listening, the positive affective and cognitive disposition toward words that we are labeling 'word consciousness' is crucial to learners' success in expanding the breadth and depth of their word knowledge over the course of their lifetimes" (Graves & Watts-Taffe, 2002, p. 145).

There are several ways to aid the development of word consciousness in students: (1) encouraging them to pay attention to the way authors choose words to communicate certain meanings, (2) promoting word play, (3) involving students in researching a word's origin or history, and (4) engaging them to search a word's usage in their everyday lives (Armbruster et al., 2001).

VOCABULARY INSTRUCTION FOR STUDENTS WHO ARE DEAF OR HARD OF HEARING

The most omnipresent aspect of deafness is its adverse effect on aural and oral language acquisition. Most children who are deaf or hard of hearing experience significant auditory and oral language delay and have smaller vocabularies than their hearing peers even with use of amplification, sign language, and special intervention (Paul, 2001).

For many students who are deaf or hard of hearing and who use American Sign Language (ASL) or other signing systems for communication, *sign vocabulary* (i.e., the words we use or recognize in signing) is used instead of or along with oral vocabulary. Sign vocabulary includes **receptive sign vocabulary** (i.e., the words we need to know to understand the signs we see) and **expressive sign vocabulary** (i.e., the words we use when we sign). However, the syntax of ASL does not correspond to English word order and its vocabulary is organized differently, incurring additional effort of forging a relationship between the two languages (see also the discussion in Chapter 1). The development of signed and spoken vocabulary for students who are deaf or hard of hearing is directly related to their success in reading (see further discussion on the link between a face-to-face language and the printed text in Chapter 7, as well as the discussion of process drama in Chapter 8).

Typically, hearing children who enter school bring a fully intact language system, including concept knowledge, to beginning reading instruction. They are able to use their knowledge of language and familiar words and meanings as a bridge to understanding print. Because of their reduced access to auditory and oral language, children who are deaf and hard of hearing typically bring a partial and still evolving language system and an impoverished vocabulary to early reading instruction. In essence, they must learn the basis of the auditory and oral language and learn to read the language at the same time (Paul, 2001). Given the significant language delays typically associated with deafness, a review of the research conducted on vocabulary instruction and acquisition for this population of students may reveal interesting findings and conclusions.

Research on Vocabulary Instruction for Students Who Are Deaf or Hard of Hearing

In their review of the research for readers who are deaf or hard of hearing and subsequent comparison with National Reading Panel findings, Schirmer and McGough (2005) and Luckner and his colleagues (Luckner, Sebald, Cooney, Young, & Goodwin Muir, 2005/2006) drew similar conclusions. Both direct and indirect instruction appears to contribute to vocabulary learning for students who are deaf or hard of hearing, though the paucity of quality research does not allow for definitive claims regarding any specific methods.

The body of research on teaching vocabulary to students who are deaf or hard of hearing is primarily focused on comparing the vocabulary knowledge of students who are deaf or hard of hearing with that of hearing counterparts (MacGinitie, 1969; Paul, 1984; Paul & Gustafson, 1991; Paul, Stallman, & O'Rourke, 1990; Walter, 1978). It is not surprising that the general finding of this line of research shows that the vocabulary knowledge of students who are deaf or hard of hearing is quantitatively reduced compared with their hearing peers, and the gap appears to increase as the frequent usage of the words decreases, particularly for multimeaning words. A few empirical studies supported the positive relationship between vocabulary knowledge and reading comprehension in deaf readers (Garrison, Long, & Dowaliby, 1997; Kelly, 1996; LaSasso & Davey, 1987).

Another line of research on vocabulary knowledge of students who are deaf or hard of hearing involves investigating the factors influencing the difficulties of a word—for example, multiplicity of meanings (Paul, 1984; Paul & Gustafson, 1991), word frequency (Walter, 1978), and context surrounding the word

(Ahn, 1996; de Villiers & Pomerantz, 1992; MacGinitie, 1969; Nolen & Wilbur, 1985; Robbins & Hatcher, 1981). In addition, there have been a few research studies of general vocabulary knowledge of readers who are deaf or hard of hearing (Fischler, 1985; Silverman-Dresner & Guilfoyle, 1972).

Intervention studies on vocabulary knowledge for students who are deaf or hard of hearing are limited. Some of them are simply descriptions of particular instructional programs without any comparison groups or sufficient information regarding their interventions. For example, Johnson and Roberson's (1988) experiment reported the number of words added to the deaf children's vocabulary after a language experience intervention; however, no comparative data were included to evaluate the significance of the intervention. Indirect instruction through rich and explicit context appears to show some promise in assisting students' vocabulary learning (de Villiers & Pomerantz, 1992). Research studies also support the direct vocabulary instruction through computer-based technology (Barker, 2003; MacGregor & Thomas, 1988; Prinz, 1991; Prinz & Nelson, 1985; Prinz, Nelson, & Stedt, 1982;Prinz, Pemberton, & Nelson, 1985).

From the available research on vocabulary learning of students who are deaf or hard of hearing, an observable pattern is the positive benefit of matching print words with signs or sign print (Schimmel, Edwards, & Prickett, 1999; Soderbergh, 1985; Suzuki & Notoya, 1984). In Koskinen and colleagues' (Koskinen, Wilson, & Jensema, 1986) intervention research, high school students who are deaf or hard of hearing showed greater retention of sight vocabulary in lessons using closed-captioned television than in lessons using traditional reading materials.

In essence, studies of vocabulary knowledge of students who are deaf or hard of hearing are mainly comparison studies on the quantitative differences between deaf readers and their hearing peers in terms of word knowledge and correlation studies on factors influencing the difficulties of a word for deaf readers. There are very few high-quality intervention studies on improving deaf students' vocabulary knowledge through instruction, particularly studies investigating the use of the strategies recommended by the National Reading Panel (2000). However, the use of instruction through rich and explicit context and multimedia methods including integrating computer-based technology, matching print with signs or sign print, and the addition of video background to the print shows some promise.

How Vocabulary Instruction Is Different for Students Who Are Deaf or Hard of Hearing

Generally speaking, the conclusions of National Reading Panel (2000) on vocabulary instruction are valid for students who are deaf or hard of hearing. However, other than the panel's general guidelines, because of their incomplete and still evolving language system and a deprived vocabulary, what kind of words should be specifically taught to students who are deaf or hard of hearing?

There are two major classifications of words in English: content words and function words. **Content words** are nouns, verbs, adjectives, and most adverbs that have a definable meaning. These words are usually labels that represent one's understanding of things or actions (*cat, eat*) or have a perceptible referent (*wet, sad, red*). **Function words** include determiners (*the, a, an*), prepositions (*near, on, over*), conjunctions (*and, but*), pronouns (*it, he, she, that, they*), and auxiliary verbs and copulas (*can, is, would*), and so on. Function words, on the other hand, have little lexical meaning or

have ambiguous meaning, but are important components of the English language. However, they create meaning units within a sentence to express grammatical relationships. Function words are common in texts, although there are far fewer of them than content words. Function words play a significant role in comprehending sentences; without them, the meaning of most sentences would be altered. For example, if we extract all the function words from the sentence *He kissed her by the house*, it becomes *kissed house*.

Typically, most speakers of a language learn function words without difficulty. Children begin the acquisition of function words in the early stages of language development through oral language. When they see these functions words in print, children have most likely heard and used these words thousands of times. However, these function words are much more difficult to learn and generalize for children who are deaf or hard of hearing for several reasons: (1) These words are generally unstressed in spoken language so most children who are deaf and many who are hard of hearing do not hear them, (2) many of the function words do not exist in ASL, (3) many of them are often omitted in other sign language systems, and (4) because function words often do not carry intonational emphasis or stress, they are also frequently contracted (as with the auxiliary *have* in *I've done*), which obscures their identification even more (Weber, 2006). To further complicate the acquisition of these words, many function words have many different uses. For example, in the sentence *In five minutes there will be a speech in the library in honor of the president*, the word *in* is used temporally (*In five minutes*), locatively (*in the library*), and to indicate purpose (*in honor of*). To make sense of this sentence, all three meanings must be inferred (see further discussion in Wang, Kretschmer, & Hartman, 2008).

Singleton, Morgan, DiGello, Wiles, and Rivers (2004) analyzed writing samples from 72 elementary school students who are deaf or hard of hearing of varied sign language proficiency and found significantly lower use of function words as compared to their hearing peers. Addressing vocabulary instruction with children who are deaf and hard of hearing must take into account that it involves teaching not only content words, but also the function words that provide the semantic and grammatical connections between them. This essentially amounts to teaching language while teaching students to read at the same time. The additional burden imposed by simultaneous language and reading instruction obviously contributes to the quantitative delays in reading vocabulary typically exhibited by this population of students (Wang, Kretschmer, & Hartman, 2008).

ASSESSMENTS OF VOCABULARY

As discussed in Chapters 4 and 5, an online database of reading assessments for students in kindergarten to second grade is available through the Southwest Educational Development Laboratory (2007). For this chapter on vocabulary, a search of tests assessing language competence was conducted. This search yielded criterion-referenced and norm-referenced assessments. The names of the assessments, copyright, publisher, and Web site for each are summarized in Tables 6-1 and 6-2. Using assessments such as these should assist teachers in understanding students' present levels of performance in the area of vocabulary and assist in developing appropriate annual goals and objectives. As discussed in Chapters 4 and 5, it is important for test administrators to review each subtest carefully to determine the effects of various administrative procedures to ensure that valid results are obtained.

INSTRUCTIONAL GOALS AND OBJECTIVES

As discussed in both Chapters 4 and 5, writing instructional goals and objectives to include in students' Individualized Education Programs is an integral part of a special educator's job. Annually, teachers are required to write a present level of performance that summarizes the results of both formal and informal assessments as well as information collected through observations of student performance. After a thorough examination of a student's skill in a particular area, the teacher must determine what can be reasonably accomplished given one year of instruction and describe an instructional goal in measurable terms. Once an acceptable goal has been established, short-term objectives or benchmarks can be written to determine distinctive, instructional elements. Table 6-3 includes a sample annual goal and objectives to address a need in the area of vocabulary. This sample instructional goal was written to address the vocabulary needs of Carlos, the student who is the subject of Case Study C. For further information regarding Carlos, please refer to the information provided in the case study section of the text.

VOCABULARY INSTRUCTION

In Chapters 4 and 5 of this text, we reviewed *A Consumer's Guide to Evaluating a Core Reading Program, Grades K–3: A Critical Elements Analysis* (Simmons & Kame'enui, 2003) to examine the elements of commercially available curricula for reading instruction for students in kindergarten through third grade. This guide, recommended by the American Federation of Teachers [AFT], was utilized by the Oregon Reading First Center (2004) to

TABLE 6-1 Norm-Referenced Assessments of Vocabulary

Name of Assessment	Copyright	Publisher	Web Site
Assessment of Literacy and Language (ALL)	2005	The Psychological Corporation	http://psychcorp.com/
Brigance Diagnostic Comprehensive Inventory of Basic Skills Revised (CIBS-R)	1999	Curriculum Associates	http://www.curriculumassociates.com/
Gates-MacGinitie Reading Tests, 4th edition (GMRT-4)	2002	Riverside Publishing Company	http://www.riverpub.com/
Group Reading Assessment and Diagnostic Evaluation (GRADE)	2001	American Guidance Service, Inc.	http://www.agsnet.com/
Kindergarten Readiness Test (KRT)	2004	Scholastic Testing Service	http://www.ststesting.com/
Metropolitan Achievement Tests Reading Diagnostic Tests 8th Edition (MAT-8)	2002	The Psychological Corporation	http://psychcorp.com/
Oral and Written Language Scales (OWLS)	1995	American Guidance Service, Inc.	http://www.agsnet.com/
Preschool Language Scale, 4th edition (PLS-4)	2002	The Psychological Corporation	http://psychcorp.com/
School Readiness Test (SRT)	2004	Scholastic Testing Service	http://www.ststesting.com/
Stanford Achievement Test, 10th edition (SAT-10)	2004	Harcourt Assessment	http://www.harcourtassessment.com/
Stanford Diagnostic Reading Test, 4th edition (SDRT-4)	2005	Harcourt Assessment	http://www.harcourtassessment.com/
Stanford Reading First	2004	Harcourt Assessment	http://www.harcourtassessment.com/
Test of Early Language Development, 3rd edition (TELD-3)	1999	ProEd Publishing	http://www.proedinc.com/
Wechsler Individual Achievement Test, 2nd edition (WIAT-II)	2005	The Psychological Corporation	http://www.txreadinginstruments.com/

TABLE 6-2 Criterion-Referenced Assessments of Vocabulary

Name of Assessment	Copyright	Publisher	Web Site
Bader Reading and Language Inventory, 5th edition	2005	Pearson Education	http://www.prenhall.com/
Ekwall/Shanker Reading Inventory, 4th edition (ESRI-4)	2000	Pearson/Allyn & Bacon	http://www.ablongman.com/
Process Assessment of the Learner (PAL) Test Battery for Reading and Writing	2001	The Psychological Corporation	http://psychcorp.com/
Reading Inventory for the Classroom, 5th edition (RIC)	2004	Pearson Education	http://www.prenhall.com/
Stieglitz Informal Reading Inventory, 3rd edition	2002	Pearson/Allyn & Bacon	http://www.ablongman.com/
Texas Primary Reading Inventory	2005	Texas Education Agency	http://www.txreadinginstruments.com/

TABLE 6-3 Annual Goal and Short-Term Objectives for Vocabulary

Area of Need: Vocabulary

Present Level of Performance:

Several subtests of the Wechsler Individual Achievement Test-II (WIAT-II) were recently administered to Carlos to gauge his level of reading achievement in several areas. Relative to vocabulary, Carlos's standard scores indicate performance that is slightly below the average of 100. Specifically, his score in the area of listening comprehension was 91, oral expression 82 and reading comprehension 75. The fact that Carlos is bilingual cannot be overlooked; therefore, a measure of English-language proficiency was also administered. Results of this assessment indicate that his scores fall slightly below the mean of 50, with his percentile in vocabulary being the weakest (24th percentile). These scores are reflective of Carlos's performance in the classroom. Carlos has difficulty comprehending passages because he lacks basic knowledge of vocabulary and struggles with providing definitions or explanations of many words. Carlos benefits greatly from having vocabulary pretaught and for opportunities to engage in extended discussions regarding key terms. Carlos is reluctant to independently attempt assignments that contain vocabulary tasks and often relies heavily on receiving support in the resource room. Because the time available to receive these services is limited, many of Carlos's assignments are incomplete or poorly done due to his lack of independence. Since enrolling in the American Sign Language course, Carlos's interest in learning new sign vocabulary has greatly increased.

Goal:

Before seeking assistance from an adult, Carlos will apply vocabulary strategies taught to attempt to identify unknown vocabulary independently in 9 out of 10 situations.

How will progress toward this goal be measured?

Teacher observation, review of assignments, student reports

Short-Term Objectives or Benchmarks Including Criteria for Evaluation

- Given a selected passage, Carlos will independently read the selection and identify any unknown words in 9 out of 10 situations.

- Given instruction in prefixes, suffixes, and root words, Carlos will independently apply this knowledge to gain meaning of unknown words in 9 out of 10 situations.

- Given instruction in using the dictionary and thesaurus, Carlos will independently utilize these reference aids to gain meaning of unknown words in 9 out of 10 situations.

- Given instruction in applying context clues to derive meaning of unknown vocabulary, Carlos will independently apply these strategies to gain meaning of unknown words in 9 out of 10 situations.

- When attempts to derive meanings of unknown vocabulary fail, Carlos will independently seek assistance from an adult in 9 out of 10 situations.

Progress Toward Annual Goal

Date	Progress*	Comments:

*Minimal (M) = anticipate that the goal will not be met by the end of the quarter
Proficient (P) = anticipate that the goal will be met by the end of the quarter
Advanced (A) = anticipate that the goal will be exceeded by the end of the quarter

evaluate nine different core reading programs. According to the checklist provided in the review, vocabulary was not considered a critical element of instruction for students at these grade levels; therefore, ratings like those included in Chapters 4 and 5 were unavailable for this chapter.

The fact that reading vocabulary was not considered an essential instructional element for students at the kindergarten through third-grade level further supports the focus of Chall's (1996) Stages 1 and 2. Beginning reading instruction for students at this level should emphasize the direct teaching of letter–sound relationships and activities that foster the development of automaticity and fluency. However, we do agree with Chall's recommendation that adults should continue to read to students to expand and enhance listening and speaking vocabularies to prepare students for the transition to Stage 3 reading.

Although vocabulary was not a focus of the comprehensive curricula review, the Oregon Reading First Center (2004) did publish a report titled *Review of Supplemental and Intervention Reading Programs*. This report represents a review of literally hundreds of curricular programs focused on the development of beginning reading skills. A copy of the full report is available online. For this chapter's focus on vocabulary, the item analysis data for vocabulary for each curriculum reviewed is available at the Oregon Reading First Center (http://oregonreadingfirst.uoregon.edu). In addition, the AFT also recommends that teachers explore the What Works Clearinghouse (http://ies.ed.gov/ncee/wwc/) and the Florida Center for Reading Research (http://www.fcrr.org) for information regarding effective interventions and instructional strategies aimed at improving vocabulary.

As with phonemic awareness and phonics instruction in Chapter 4 and fluency instruction in Chapter 5, we encourage readers to explore the resources provided above to identify successful vocabulary interventions to implement with students who are deaf or hard of hearing. In addition to published reading curriculums, many print and online resources are available to provide teachers with ideas for implementing effective vocabulary instruction in the classrooms. A list of these teacher resources is included at the end of this chapter. In addition, teacher-created materials may also be used to address vocabulary instruction. A description of several activities is provided in the following section.

Vocabulary Instructional Activities

The National Reading Panel (2000) recommended two general instructional strategies to promote vocabulary growth for students: specific word instruction and word-learning strategies. As discussed earlier in this chapter, it is impossible to directly teach all the words students will need to know; therefore, teachers should consider teaching important, useful, and difficult words. For students who are deaf or hard of hearing, teachers should also take into account function words because these words are generally unstressed in spoken language, many of them do not exist in ASL, they are often omitted in other sign language systems, and the meaning of these words can vary based on the content. To promote vocabulary acquisition, the National Reading Panel suggested that specific words be taught prior to being encountered in text, extended instruction be provided to promote active engagement with vocabulary, and repeated exposures to vocabulary in various contexts be offered to foster increased knowledge of words. In light of the National Reading Panel's recommendations, the following sample activities are offered.

- *Word Pyramid:* This activity is an engaging way for students to familiarize themselves with new vocabulary. Students can work individually, with partners, or in small groups to complete this activity. The instructional arrangement will depend on the number of words and number of students in the class. The activity begins with the teacher supplying a copy of a blank word pyramid (see Figure 6-1) and a word for students to investigate. Using a dictionary and thesaurus, students explore their word, complete the word pyramid, and then present it to the class. This activity

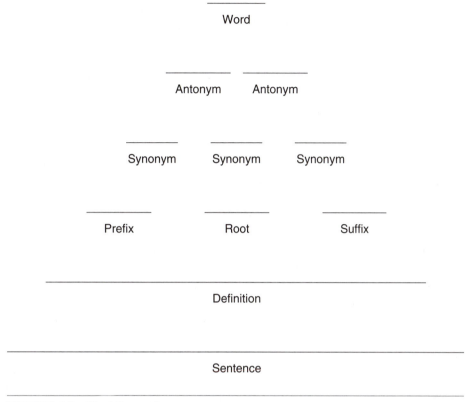

FIGURE 6-1 *Word Pyramid*

is particularly useful when beginning a new unit of study. The completed word pyramids can then be posted in the classroom to serve as a reference for students. This activity can be easily modified to meet the age and skill level of students. For example, with younger students, portions of the pyramid can be removed (e.g., prefix, root, suffix) and items such as drawing a picture added. Students can also create a vocabulary collage using pictures from magazines to creatively illustrate the various levels of the word pyramid. Additional graphic organizers such as vocabulary webs or trees can also be used in place of the pyramid design.

- *Word Play:* This activity is an excellent way to actively engage students in learning the meanings of new words prior to reading a selection. In this charade-like activity, students are divided into teams and given a word. The goal is to create a one-minute skit that dramatizes the meaning of the word without using the actual word. A "silent movie" format can also be used in this activity to ensure that students do not include the word in their dramatization. Teams can then compete to see how many words they can guess. This activity can also be a great way to review vocabulary at the end of a unit or after completing a novel.

- *Vocabulary Crossword:* Creating crossword puzzles allows teachers to provide repeated exposures to vocabulary in various contexts. Teachers can vary the clues offered in the puzzle depending on the students' knowledge of the word. For example, when first introducing a word, the exact definition presented in class may be used to complete the puzzle. However, once students have gained knowledge and insight into the meaning of the word, the puzzle can expose them to the word in a different context. The teacher has the option to supply a word bank as well. Students can also be asked to create their own puzzles in order to indicate their knowledge of the new vocabulary taught. Several online resources are available for creating crossword puzzles. Crossword Puzzle Games (http://www.crosswordpuzzlegames.com) is a nice source.

Conclusion

This chapter focused on the importance of vocabulary instruction for children and adolescents who are deaf or hard of hearing. The recommendations of the National Reading Panel (2000) and a synthesis of the available research on individuals who are deaf or hard of hearing were the primary sources used to guide this discussion. Scientific research on vocabulary instruction concludes that although some vocabulary must be taught directly, the majority of vocabulary is learned indirectly. Suggestions on facilitating children's indirect vocabulary learning and guidance on direct vocabulary instruction are provided. The majority of students who are deaf or hard of hearing experience significant auditory or oral language delay and have smaller vocabularies than their hearing peers even with use of amplification, sign language, and special intervention. For the many students who are deaf or hard of hearing who use sign language as their primary form of communication, sign vocabulary is used instead of or along with oral vocabulary. Sign vocabulary includes both receptive and expressive skills. Schirmer and McGough (2005) and Luckner and his colleagues (Luckner et al., 2005/2006) drew similar conclusions regarding vocabulary instruction for students who are deaf or hard of hearing. Both direct and indirect instruction appears to contribute to vocabulary learning for students who are deaf or hard of hearing; however, the lack of quality research conducted in this area makes it difficult to recommend specific instructional methods. Some potential effective teaching strategies for vocabulary instruction of students who are deaf or hard of hearing are presented. Furthermore, special attention should be paid to direct instruction of function words for students who are deaf or hard of hearing.

Chapter Summary

- Vocabulary refers to the words we must know to comprehend and communicate effectively. There are four different types of vocabulary: listening, speaking, reading vocabulary, and writing vocabulary. Vocabulary knowledge contributes greatly to the ability to comprehend text and general school success.

- Children acquire vocabulary indirectly by engaging in oral language, listening to adults read to them, and reading extensively on their own. Direct vocabulary instruction should focus on specific word instruction and teach word-learning strategies. In addition, teachers need to foster word consciousness to deepen and expand students' vocabulary knowledge.

- For students who are deaf or hard of hearing, vocabulary instruction that integrates rich and explicit context and multimedia methods including integrating computer-based technology, matching print with signs or sign print, and adding

video background to the print shows some promise.

- In addition to content words, teachers of students who are deaf or hard of hearing must take into account the difficulty of English function words when planning vocabulary instruction.

REVIEW QUESTIONS

1. According to National Reading Panel (2000), what are the two ways students acquire new vocabulary?

2. What instructional methods should teachers employ in direct vocabulary instruction?

3. How does the definition of vocabulary differ for students who are deaf or hard hearing and who utilize sign language for communication?

4. What are the general conclusions of the research related to vocabulary for students who are deaf or hard of hearing?

5. Why do English function words pose a particular challenge for students who are deaf or hard of hearing?

REFLECTIVE QUESTIONS

1. Using the examples provided in this chapter as your guide, create two instructional activities that can be used to directly teach content vocabulary to students who are deaf of hard of hearing.

2. What strategies would you recommend to a parent of a child who is deaf or hard of hearing to promote indirect vocabulary acquisition at home?

APPLICATION EXERCISES

1. Using the annual goal and objective presented in this chapter, write a week-long lesson plan to address one of the short-term objectives written for Carlos.

2. Write a present level of performance, an annual goal, and at least three short-term objectives to address the vocabulary needs of Aidan, the subject of Case Study A.

SUGGESTED READINGS AND RESOURCES

Readings

Baumann, J. F., & Kame'enui, E. J. (2003). *Vocabulary instruction: Research to practice (solving problems in teaching of literacy)*. New York: Guilford Press.

Bear, D. R., Invemizzi, M., Templeton, S. R., & Johnston, F. (2007). *Words their way: Word study for phonics, vocabulary, and spelling instruction*. (4th ed.). Upper Saddle Ridge, NJ: Prentice Hall.

Beck, I. L., McKeown, M. G., & Kucan, L. (2002). *Bringing words to life: Robust vocabulary instruction*. New York: Guilford Press.

Blachowicz, C., & Fischer, P. J. (2005). *Teaching vocabulary in all classrooms*. (3rd ed.). Upper Saddle Ridge, NJ: Prentice Hall.

Blanchfield, C. L., & Tompkins, G. E. (2003). *Teaching vocabulary: Fifty creative strategies, K-12*. Upper Saddle Ridge, NJ: Prentice Hall.

Nickelson, L. (1999). *Quick activities to build a very voluminous vocabulary (Grades 4–8)*. New York: Scholastic Professional Books.

Hiebert, E. H., & Kamil, M. L. (2005). *Teaching and learning vocabulary: Bringing research to practice*. Mahwah, NJ: Lawrence Erlbaum.

Resources

Lesson Plan Central
http://lessonplancentral.com/lessons/Language_Arts/Vocabulary/index.htm

Vocabulary Instruction
http://www.literacy.uconn.edu/compre.htm#vocab

Vocabulary University
http://www.vocabulary.com/

Word Study
http://davis.dadecountyschools.org/wordstudy/

www.TechTeachers.com
http://www.techteachers.com/vocabulary.htm

REFERENCES

Ahn, S. (1996). *A study of incidental vocabulary learning by students with hearing impairment*. Unpublished doctoral dissertation, Ohio State University, Columbus, Ohio.

Armbruster, B. B., Lehr, F., & Osborn, J. (2001). *Put reading first: The research building blocks for teaching children to read kindergarten through grade three*. Jessup, MD: National Institute for Literacy.

Barker, L. J. (2003). Computer-assisted vocabulary acquisition: The CSLU vocabulary tutor in oral-deaf education. *Journal of Deaf Studies and Deaf Education, 8* (2), 187–198.

Carnine, D. W., Silbert, J., Kame'enui, E. J., & Tarver, S. G. (2004). *Direct instruction reading*. (4th ed.). Upper Saddle River, NJ: Pearson Education.

Carnine, D. W., Silbert, J., Kame'enui, E. J., Tarver, S. G., & Jungjohann, K. (2004). *Teaching struggling and at-risk readers—A direct instruction approach*. Upper Saddle River, NJ: Pearson Education.

Chall, J. S. (1996). *Stages of reading development*. (2nd ed.). New York: McGraw-Hill.

de Villiers, P., & Pomerantz, S. (1992). Hearing-impaired students learning new words from written context. *Applied psycholinguistics, 13*, 409–431.

Fischler, I. (1985). Word recognition, use of context, and reading skill among deaf college students. *Reading Research Quarterly, 20*, 203–218.

Garrison, W., Long, G., & Dowaliby, F. (1997). Working memory capacity and comprehension processes in deaf readers. *Journal of Deaf Studies and Deaf Education, 2*, 78–94.

Graves, M. F., & Watts-Taffe, S. M. (2002). The place of word consciousness in a research-based vocabulary program. In A. E. Farstrup & S. J. Samuels (Eds.). *What research has to say about reading instruction* (3rd. ed). Newark, DE: International Reading Association.

Irvin, J. L. (1998). *Reading and the middle school student: Strategies to enhance literacy* (2nd ed.). Boston: Allyn & Bacon.

Johnson, M. A., & Roberson, G. F. (1988). The language experience approach: Its use with young hearing-impaired students. *American Annals of the Deaf, 133*, 223–225.

Kelly, L. (1996). The interaction of syntactic competence and vocabulary during reading by deaf students. *Journal of Deaf Studies and Deaf Education, 1*, 1, 75–90.

Koskinen, P. S., Wilson, R. M., & Jensema, C. J. (1986). Using closed-captioned television in the teaching of reading to deaf students. *American Annals of the Deaf, 131*, 43–46.

LaSasso, C., & Davey, B. (1987). The relationship between lexical knowledge and reading comprehension for prelingually, profoundly hearing-impaired students. *Volta Review, 89*, 211–220.

Luckner, J., Sebald, A. N., Cooney, J., Young, J., & Goodwin Muir, S. (2005/2006). An examination of the evidence-based literacy research in deaf education. *American Annals of the Deaf, 150* (5), 443–456.

MacGinitie, W. (1969). Flexibility if dealing with alternative meanings of words. In J. Rosenstein & W. MacGinitie (Eds.), *Verbal behavior of the deaf child: Studies of word meanings and associations* (pp. 45–55). New York: Columbia University, Teachers College Press.

MacGregor, S. K., & Thomas, L. B. (1988). A computer-mediated text system to develop communication skills for hearing-impaired students. *American Annals of the Deaf, 133* (4), 280–284.

Nagy, W. E., & Anderson, R. C. (1984). How many words are there in printed school English? *Reading Research Quarterly, 19*, 304–330.

Nagy, W. E., Anderson, R. C., & Herman, P. (1987). Learning word meanings from context during normal reading. *American Educational Research Journal, 24*, 237–270.

Nagy, W. E., Herman, P., & Anderson, R. C. (1985). Learning words from context. *Reading Research Quarterly, 20*, 233–253.

National Reading Panel (2000). *Report of the National Reading Panel: Teaching children to read—An evidence-based assessment of the scientific research literature on reading and its implications for reading instruction.* Jessup, MD: National Institute for Literacy at EDPubs.

Nolen, S., & Wilbur, R. (1985). The effects of context on deaf students' comprehension of difficult sentences. *American Annals of the Deaf, 130*, 231–235.

Oregon Reading First Center. (2004). *Review of Comprehensive Reading Programs.*

Retrieved October 21, 2007 from http://reading.uoregon.edu/curricula/intro_summ_review_3-04.pdf.

Paul, P. (1984). *The comprehension of multi-meaning words from selected frequency levels by deaf and hearing subjects.* Unpublished doctoral dissertation, University of Illinois, Urbana-Champaign.

Paul, P. (2001). *Language and deafness* (3rd ed.). San Diego: Singular Publishing Group.

Paul, P., & Gustafson, G. (1991). Hearing-impaired students' comprehension of high-frequency multimeaning words. *Remedial and Special Education, 12,* 4, 52–62.

Paul, P., Stallman, A., & O'Rourke, J. (1990). *Using three test formats to assess good and poor readers' word knowledge* (Tech. Rep. No. 509). Urbana-Champaign: University of Illinois Center for the Study of Reading.

Prinz, P. M. (1991). Literacy and language development within microcomputer-videodisc-assisted interactive contexts. *Journal of Childhood Communication Disorders, 14,* 67–80.

Prinz, P. M., & Nelson, K. E. (1985). "Alligator eats cookie": Acquisition of writing and reading skills by deaf children using the microcomputer. *Applied Psycholinguistics, 6,* 283–306.

Prinz, P. M., Nelson, K. E., & Stedt, J. D. (1982). Early reading in young deaf children using microcomputer technology. *American Annals of the Deaf, 127,* 529–535.

Prinz, P. M., Pemberton, E., & Nelson, K. E. (1985). The ALPHA interactive microcomputer system for teaching reading, writing, and communication skills to

hearing-impaired children. *American Annals of the Deaf, 130,* 444–461.

Robbins, N., & Hatcher, C. (1981). The effects of syntax on the reading comprehension of hearing-impaired children. *Volta Review, 83,* 105–115.

Schimmel, C. S., Edwards, S. G., & Prickett, H. T. (1999). Reading? … Pah! (I got it!): Innovative reading techniques for successful deaf readers. *American Annals of the Deaf, 144,* 298–308.

Schirmer, B. R., & McGough, S. M. (2005). Teaching reading to children who are deaf: Do the conclusions of the National Reading Panel apply? *Review of Educational Research, 75* (1), 83–117.

Silverman-Dresner, T., & Guilfoyle, G. (1972). *Vocabulary norms for deaf children: The Lexington school for the deaf education series, book VII.* Washington, DC: Alexander Graham Bell Association for the Deaf.

Simmons, D. C., & Kame'enui, E. J. (2003). *A consumer's guide to evaluating a core reading program, grades K-3: A critical elements analysis.* Retrieved October 21, 2007, from http://teacher.scholastic.com/products/fundingconnection/pdf/Kameenui_GR_Blue.pdf

Singleton, J. L., Morgan, D., DiGello, E., Wiles, J., & Rivers, R. (2004). Vocabulary use by low, moderate, and high ASL-proficient writers compared to hearing ESL and monolingual speakers. *Journal of Deaf Studies and Deaf Education, 9* (1), 86–103.

Snow, C. E., Griffin, P., & Burns, M. S. (Eds.) (2005). *Knowledge to support the teaching of reading: Preparing teachers for a changing world.* San Francisco: John Wiley & Sons.

Soderbergh, R. (1985). Early reading with deaf children. *Quarterly Review of Education, 15*, 77–85.

Southwest Educational Development Laboratory. (2007). *Reading assessment database.* Retrieved March 3, 2007, from http://www.sedl.org/reading/rad/database.html.

Stahl, S., & Nagy, W. (2006). *Teaching word meanings.* Mahwah, NJ: Erlbaum.

Suzuki, S., & Notoya, M. (1984). Teaching written language to deaf infants and preschoolers. *Topics in Early Childhood Special Education, 3* (4), 10–16.

Walter, G. (1978). Lexical abilities of hearing and hearing-impaired children. *American Annals of the Deaf, 123*, 976–982.

Wang, Y., Kretschmer, R. & Hartman, M. (2008). Reading and students who are d/Deaf or hard of hearing. *Journal of Balanced Reading Instruction, 15* (2), 53–68.

Weber, R. (2006). Function words in the prosody of fluent reading. *Journal of Reading Research, 29* (3), 258–269.

CHAPTER 7

COMPREHENSION

Spoken language and reading have much in common. If the printed words can be efficiently recognized, comprehension of connected text depends heavily on the reader's oral-language abilities, particularly with regard to understanding the meanings of words that have been identified and the syntactic and semantic relationships among them. Indeed, many early research reports called attention to the differences between good and poor readers in their comprehension and production of structural relations within spoken sentences (Snow, Burns, & Griffin, 1998, p. 108).

CHAPTER OBJECTIVES

After completing this chapter, the reader will be able to:

- Describe the National Reading Panel's findings relative to comprehension instruction

- Explain the research exploring the efficacy of comprehension instruction with students who are deaf or hard of hearing

- Discuss appropriate Individualized Education Program (IEP) goals and short-term objectives for comprehension instruction

- Create instructional activities to teach comprehension

- Describe Bloom's Taxonomy and the Core Knowledge Curriculum

INTRODUCTION

Reading comprehension is a complicated cognitive activity involving numerous skills and strategies. However, the famous Durkin (1978) study, What Classroom Observations Reveal About Reading Comprehension Instruction, found that the actual time devoted to comprehension instruction accounted for a mere 2% of the typical reading instructional session. In the past 30 years, we have learned much about both the process of reading comprehension and about effective reading comprehension instruction, which have been grounded mainly in studies of good readers.

The findings of the National Reading Panel (2000) and a review of research on good readers' comprehension habits (Duke & Pearson, 2003) illustrate that good readers are purposeful and active. That is, good readers have clear goals (i.e., purpose) during reading—for example, learning a recipe to make apple pie, finding out how to get to the museum using a guidebook, or experiencing pleasure reading classic literature. They constantly evaluate whether their goals are being met as they read the text. Before they read, good readers normally skim through the text looking for information that might be most relevant to their reading goals—for example, the structure of the text or text sections. Good readers find reading satisfying and productive.

Meanwhile, good readers actively make sense of the text. They frequently formulate predictions as they read and they read selectively (i.e., knowing what to read, what to read thoroughly, what to skip, what to reread, and so on). Good readers constantly construct, revise, and question the meanings they make during reading. They know when they understand or do not understand, and they know how to deal with the gaps using their prior knowledge of the world, their knowledge of vocabulary, language structure, and genre, as well as their knowledge of reading strategies and plans. While they read, good readers keep the information regarding authors of the text in mind such as their style, historical background, beliefs, intentions, and so on. In addition, "[f]or good readers, text processing occurs not only during 'reading' as we have traditionally defined it, but also during short breaks taken during reading, even after the 'reading' itself has commenced, even after the 'reading' has ceased" (Duke & Pearson, 2003, p. 206).

In this chapter, the National Reading Panel's (2000) conclusions and suggestions for instruction in the area of reading comprehension are described in greater detail. Studies are also reviewed that have explored the efficacy of using these reading comprehension instructional techniques with students who are deaf or hard of hearing. Guidelines for implementing comprehension instruction with students are discussed, and an overview of several assessments of reading comprehension is supplied. A sample Individualized Education Program (IEP) goal and objectives to address reading comprehension needs are provided. Evaluations of selected reading comprehension curricula that incorporate comprehension instruction as well as sample comprehension instructional activities are included. An overview of Bloom's Taxonomy and the Core Knowledge Curriculum is also provided. In the conclusion, major points are highlighted, and directions for future research are discussed.

COMPREHENSION

What is reading comprehension? As discussed in Chapter 1, there have been various definitions of reading comprehension. We adopt the definition from Vellutino (2003) for the discussion in this chapter:

> Reading comprehension may be simply defined as the ability to obtain meaning from written text for some purpose. It is a complex process that depends on adequate development of two component processes: word recognition and language comprehension. Word recognition is the process whereby the individual visually recognizes a particular array of letters as a familiar word and retrieves the name and meaning of that word from memory. Language comprehension is the process whereby the individual is able to understand and relate the meanings of words and sentences encountered in spoken and written text, and combine them in ways that allow understanding of the broader concepts and ideas represented by those words and sentences. (p. 51)

Reading is a complicated process that develops over time. Fluent word recognition is a basic prerequisite for adequate reading comprehension, although it is by no means sufficient for skilled comprehension. Both adequate word recognition and advanced development of language comprehension and knowledge-acquisition skills are components of proficient comprehension. According to Chall (1996), using reading to learn subject matter does not occur until students have learned to read. However, teachers should emphasize reading comprehension from the beginning in the primary grades instead of waiting until students have mastered "the basics of reading"—that is, word recognition and fluency. Reading comprehension instruction should be emphasized at all grade levels.

The National Reading Panel (2000) concluded that students can be taught to improve their reading comprehension by using specific cognitive strategies or by reasoning strategically when they encounter barriers to understanding the texts that they are reading. Informal acquisition of these strategies happens to some extent, whereas explicit or formal instruction in the application of comprehension strategies has been found to be highly effective in improving understanding. Before students become purposeful and active readers who are in control of their own reading comprehension, they typically require teachers' demonstrations of comprehension strategies.

Effective Strategies for Improving Text Comprehension

The National Reading Panel (2000) suggested six strategies that appear to have a solid scientific basis for enhancing text comprehension: (1) monitoring comprehension, (2) using graphic and semantic organizers, (3) answering questions, (4) generating questions, (5) recognizing story structure, and (6) summarizing. Some of these strategies are effective when used alone; others are more valuable when used as part of a multiple-strategy technique. A brief description of each instructional strategy is provided in the following sections.

Monitoring Comprehension

Readers who are aware of when they understand what they read and when they do not and then utilize the appropriate strategies to fix the arising problems in their understanding are utilizing *comprehension-monitoring* strategies. Comprehension monitoring is a critical part of metacognition. *Metacognition* refers to "thinking about thinking." Metacognitive strategies are employed by good readers to think about and maintain control over their reading. For example, using comprehension monitoring, a good reader may clarify the purpose of reading and preview the text before reading; examine their understanding, modifying his reading speed to correspond to the difficulty of the text and "fixing up" evolving comprehension problems during reading, and, finally, verifying his understanding of the text afterward (Armbruster, Lehr, & Osborn, 2001).

The National Reading Panel (2000) identified the following effective comprehension-monitoring strategies for the effective reader: (1) identifying where the difficulty arises, (2) identifying what the difficulty is, (3) reiterating the difficult sentence or passage using his own words, (4) looking back through the text, and (5) looking forward in the text for information that might assist him in resolving the difficulty.

Using Graphic and Semantic Organizers

Graphic organizers—which are also known as *maps, webs, charts, graphs, frames,* and *clusters*—use diagrams or other pictorial devices to illustrate concepts and interrelationships among concepts in a text. **Semantic organizers**—which are also referred to as *semantic maps* and *semantic webs*—are graphic organizers that look similar to a spider web—that is, lines connect a central concept to various related ideas and events.

With informational text in the content areas such as science and social studies textbooks as well as trade books, graphic organizers can help students understand how concepts fit common text structures. With narrative text, graphic organizers can assist students learn the story structure as story maps. The National Reading Panel (2000) concluded that the advantages of using graphic organizers include

(1) helping students concentrate on text structure during reading, (2) offering students practical tools to investigate and visually represent relationship in a text, and (3) assisting students in writing well-organized text summaries.

Answering Questions

Answering questions posed by the teacher has been shown to strongly support and advance students' learning from reading. These questions provide students with a purpose for reading and help students focus on what they are to learn. According to the National Reading Panel (2000), teacher questioning encourages students to think actively and monitor their comprehension during reading. Furthermore, teacher questioning assists students in reviewing content and relating what they have learned to what they already know.

There are two types of question-answering instruction: One teaches students to go back to the text to find answers to questions that they cannot answer after the initial reading, whereas the other helps students understand question-answer relationships—that is, the relationships between questions and where the answers can be found. There are three different question-answer relationships: (1) text explicit (i.e., information is stated explicitly in one sentence), (2) text implicit (i.e., information is implied in two or more sentences), and (3) scriptal (i.e., information cannot be found in the text at all but from part of the reader's prior knowledge or experience) (Armbruster et al., 2001).

Generating Questions

Generating questions is a higher level of reading strategy than answering questions. The report of the National Reading Panel (2000) reveals that by asking their own questions, students can be actively aware of whether they can answer the questions and whether they understand the text. In particular, students can learn to generate questions that require them to integrate information from different segments of the text. As discussed previously in this text, generating questions is one of the most important skills for developing a critical reader stance. This activity can be conducted for one passage or across several passages (e.g., see discussions in Paris & Stahl, 2005).

Recognizing Story Structure

Story structure is the way in which the content and events of a story are organized into a plot. A better understanding of the story structure can result in greater appreciation, understanding, and memory for stories. Story structure instruction is typically not used for informational text or poetry. Using story maps to show the sequence of events in simple stories is a common strategy in recognizing story structure. Story structure instruction emphasizes two basic skills: (1) identifying the categories of content—for example, setting, initiating events, internal reactions, goals, attempts, and outcomes; and (2) understanding how this content is organized into a plot (Armbruster et al., 2001).

Summarizing

A summary refers to a synthesis of the important ideas in a text. Instruction in *summarizing* helps students to determine and connect main ideas, reduce redundant and unnecessary information, and remember what they read. The National Reading Panel (2000) recommends that instruction in summarizing include teaching students to (1) identify or generate what is important in the text, (2) condense the

information, and (3) restate it using their own words.

Guidelines for Teaching Comprehension Strategies

The members of the National Reading Panel (2000) not only identified six effective comprehension strategies but also offered three guidelines for how to teach these comprehension strategies. The panel concluded that effective comprehension strategy instruction (1) is explicit or direct, (2) can be accomplished through cooperative learning, and (3) helps readers use comprehension strategies flexibly and in combination with one another. A brief overview of each instructional method is supplied in the following sections.

Explicit or Direct Instruction

In explicit instruction, teachers directly tell students why and when they should use particular strategies and how to apply them. Explicit teaching approaches are shown to be most effective. The four steps of explicit instruction recommended by the National Reading Panel (2000) include (1) *direct explanation* in which the teacher explains why the strategy helps comprehension and when to apply it; (2) *modeling* in which the teacher uses "thinking aloud" to demonstrate how to apply the strategy while reading the text; (3) *guided practice* in which the teacher guides and facilitates students as they learn how and when to apply the strategy; and (4) *application* in which the teacher facilitates students practicing the strategy until they can apply it on their own. The teacher should gradually release the responsibility of comprehending the text to the students following the above four steps. This four-step teaching process, which involves gradually asking students to assuming additional responsibility for applying a skill, is often referred to as *scaffolding*.

Cooperative Learning

Cooperative learning, which is also known as *collaborative learning*, refers to the activities that require students to work together as partners or in small groups on clearly defined tasks. Students can help each other learn and apply comprehension strategies while teachers are facilitating the group efforts, providing demonstrations of the strategies, and monitoring students' progress. Cooperative learning is particularly effective in content-area subject instruction (National Reading Panel, 2000).

Use Comprehension Strategies Flexibly and in Combination

Good readers are able to use multiple strategies flexibly and coordinate them to assist their comprehension. *Reciprocal teaching* is an example of effective multiple-strategy instruction that includes (1) asking questions about what they are reading, (2) summarizing parts of the text, (3) clarifying unknown words or sentences, and (4) predicting what might happen next in the text (Armbruster et al., 2001).

Other Identified Effective Comprehension Strategy Instruction

In addition to the six strategies that have received the strongest support from research, the National Reading Panel (2000) identified two additional comprehension strategies that have received some scientific support: (1) making use of prior knowledge and (2) using mental imagery.

Prior knowledge and world experience are frequently used by good readers to assist their understanding of the text. Teachers can preview the text with the students by: 1) asking what they already know about the content, what they know about the author, and what text structure the author is likely to use; 2) discussing the key vocabulary; and 3) presenting pictures or diagrams to prepare the students for the text.

Mental pictures or images are also often used by good readers during reading. Visualizing during reading can help readers, especially younger readers, to understand and remember the text. Teachers can facilitate the students to form visual images of the text by encouraging them to picture a setting, character, or event of what they are reading.

ADDITIONAL RESEARCH ON COMPREHENSION INSTRUCTION

Duke and Pearson (2003) further propose that good practices for developing reading comprehension should be *balanced*, which means that effective comprehension instruction should include both explicitly teaching specific comprehension strategies and allowing student to actually read, write, and discuss the text during informal learning. They offer the following suggestions for creating a supportive classroom context in which comprehension strategies can be taught explicitly: (1) Explicit comprehension strategy instruction should be accompanied by plenty of time applying these strategies during actual reading; (2) students need to experience reading real texts beyond those designed exclusively for reading instruction and read them with a clear and compelling purpose in mind; (3) students should read a wide range of text genres; (4) well-chosen texts, hands-on activities, field trips, conversations, and other experiences are critical in establishing an environment rich in vocabulary and concept development; (5) students need to have substantial facility in the accurate and automatic decoding of words; (6) the connection between reading and writing should be emphasized in instruction to allow students to have plenty of time writing so they can develop their abilities to write like a reader and read like a writer; and (7) students should be immerged in an environment rich in high quality teacher-to-student and student-to-student conversations about the text (Duke & Pearson, 2003).

Comprehension Instruction for Students Who Are Deaf or Hard of Hearing

Because of the close relationship between reading comprehension and language comprehension (see the definition of reading comprehension at the beginning of this chapter) and the language deficit of most students who are deaf and many who are hard of hearing (see the discussion in Chapter 6), it is not difficult to understand the lower levels of reading comprehension compared to hearing peers. After all, language is a primary system whereas literacy is a secondary system (Snow, Griffin, & Burns, 2005). The report from *Committee on the Prevention of Reading Difficulties in Young Children* (Snow et al., 1998; see also McGuinness, 2004, 2005) concluded:

> [T]he successful reader must have skills in analyzing language in order to understand how the alphabetic code represents meaningful message. . . . Typical English-speaking children have considerable knowledge available for analysis at the time they enter school. Non-English speakers have much less basis for knowing whether their reading is correct because the crucial meaning-making process is short circuited by lack of language knowledge. Giving a child initial reading instruction in a language that he or she does not yet speak thus can undermine the child's chance to see literacy as a powerful form of communication, by knocking the support of meaning out from underneath the process of learning. (p. 237)

This is consistent with the fact that the vast majority of studies on reading comprehension for students who are deaf or hard of hearing are related to the students' knowledge of syntax, figurative language, and other language variables, which is not a major research thrust for studies on students with typical language development. There have also been some research studies on prior knowledge and metacognition (e.g., comprehension monitoring) of students who are deaf or hard of hearing (e.g., see the review in Paul, 2003). The following sections provide a review of the research on the comprehension abilities of students who are deaf or hard of hearing mainly from four areas: syntax, figurative language, prior knowledge, and metacognition. We then discuss how comprehension instruction is different for students who are deaf or hard of hearing in these four areas.

Research on Comprehension Instruction for Students Who Are Deaf or Hard of Hearing

Schirmer and McGough (2005) found concordance with the National Reading Panel (2000) findings on the general value of teaching comprehension strategies to students who are deaf or hard of hearing; however, they again note the scarcity of research in this area. Citing a few studies that addressed some of the instructional strategies investigated in the National Reading Panel review (e.g., comprehension monitoring, text structure, question answering, and question generating) and other studies investigating strategies not mentioned at all by the National Reading Panel (e.g., syntactic knowledge, background, mental imagery, and inference making), they could not make any definitive assertions on any one strategy or instructional technique in terms of reading comprehension instruction for students who are deaf or hard of hearing. In this text, we concentrate on four main areas of reading comprehension instruction for students who are deaf or hard of hearing: syntactic knowledge, figurative language, prior knowledge, and metacognition. We believe that these strategies should be emphasized for students who are deaf or hard of hearing above and beyond the recommendations of the National Reading Panel (2000).

Research on Syntactic Knowledge of Students Who Are Deaf or Hard of Hearing

Syntax refers to word order or sentence organization. Undoubtedly, syntax has been one of the most researched areas in literacy and deafness because of the obvious difficulty students who are deaf or hard of hearing experience with English syntax. For example, Miller's (2005) study of prelingually deafened children found that although they could identify many words in isolation, they lacked the syntactic knowledge necessary for proper processing of words at the sentence level. The field is heavily influenced by Chomsky's (1957, 1965, 1975, 1988) belief that syntax is critical in describing the grammar of a language and especially in comprehending the mind of the language user.

Quigley and his associates (Quigley, Power, & Steinkamp, 1977; Quigley, Smith, & Wilbur, 1974; Quigley, Wilbur, & Montanelli, 1974, 1976) have conducted extensive studies comparing the syntactic knowledge of students who are deaf or hard of hearing with that of their hearing peers. The results demonstrated quantitative delays of students who are deaf or hard of hearing in comprehending assorted syntactic structures. At the same time, the findings showed the qualitative similarities of students with and without hearing loss in terms of the stages proceeded through, the errors made, and the strategies used in comprehending these syntactic structures. Other research studies have focused on the knowledge of particular syntactic structures in students who are deaf or hard of hearing (Kelly, 1998; Lillo-Martin, Hanson, & Smith, 1992; Wilbur & Goodhart, 1985; Wilbur, Goodhart, & Fuller, 1989). Based on these studies, *Reading Milestones* (Quigley, McAnally, King, & Rose, 1991), a reading curriculum designed to control vocabulary and syntactic structures, was specifically developed to mirror the developmental sequence of deaf readers. Unfortunately, there has been no experimental research assessing the effectiveness of the series with readers who are deaf or hard of hearing.

The importance of syntactic knowledge and the role it plays in reading comprehension skill acquisition for readers who are deaf or hard of hearing has been emphasized in Quigley and his colleagues' research. However, other researchers argue that the significance of other related factors need to be explored in order to gain a better understanding of readers' English syntactic knowledge. For example, the context information (McGill-Franzen & Gormley, 1980; McKnight, 1989; Nolen & Wilbur, 1985), readers' top-down comprehension of the text (Ewoldt, 1981), text coherence

(Israelite & Helfrich, 1988), semantic issues (Miller, 2000; Stoefen-Fisher, 1987–1988; Yurkowski & Ewoldt, 1986), difficulties in lower-level phonological processing (Lillo-Martin, Hanson, & Smith, 1991, 1992), and pictorial symbols (Diebold & Waldron, 1988) are additional factors that warrant investigation for students who are deaf or hard of hearing.

In short, although the limited syntactic competence of students who are deaf or hard of hearing is not the only skill that contributes to overall reading comprehension ability, the importance of syntax should not be underestimated. As previously mentioned, most of the studies in this area are still in a stage of debate and the importance of syntactic knowledge for reading comprehension has yet to be determined in a comprehensive manner. What appears to be lacking in the field are intervention studies that will contribute to the improvement of syntactic knowledge of students who are deaf or hard of hearing, which is directly related to their language development and reading comprehension.

Research on Figurative Language of Students Who Are Deaf or Hard of Hearing

Another language issue that is closely connected with the overall reading abilities of students who are deaf or hard of hearing is **figurative language,** which includes figures of speech (e.g., fixed idioms) such as similes (*She smiles like a flower*), metaphors (*The tree is an umbrella*), and idiomatic expressions (*I ran into an old friend yesterday*). Similar to the research on students who learn English as a second language (Bernhardt, 1991), research on students who are deaf or hard of hearing (King & Quigley, 1985; Paul, 1998, 2003) has demonstrated that, besides vocabu-

lary and syntax, figurative language is another area in which many students who are deaf or hard of hearing experience difficulties, although it is almost impossible to isolate the effects of limited vocabulary and syntactic knowledge.

In comparing students who are deaf or hard of hearing with their hearing peers, research in this area (Conley, 1976; Payne & Quigley, 1987) reiterates the long-standing findings: The performance of readers who are deaf or hard of hearing on comprehension of figurative language is quantitatively reduced and barely varies across ages. Furthermore, research indicates that students' comprehension of figurative language is closely connected with their reading comprehension (Fruchter, Wilbur, & Fraser, 1984; Orlando & Shulman, 1989).

Similar to the studies of syntactic knowledge of students who are deaf or hard of hearing, many research studies on the figurative language knowledge of students have investigated performance when other language variables—for example, the vocabulary and syntax (Iran-Nejad, Ortony, & Rittenhouse, 1981)—were controlled. From a top-down framework, some researchers argued the importance of a holistic understanding of the text in students' comprehension of idioms (Wilbur, Fraser, & Fruchter, 1981).

As with syntax, a limited understanding of figurative language cannot fully explain the poor overall reading achievement of students who are deaf or hard of hearing; however, it is generally accepted that their figurative language knowledge is closely related to their reading comprehension. As with many areas in the field of literacy and deafness, there have not been innovative intervention studies aimed at improving students' figurative language knowledge.

Research on Prior Knowledge of Students Who Are Deaf or Hard of Hearing

Prior knowledge is typically categorized as (1) passage-specific prior knowledge that refers to knowledge about the language elements or text information and (2) topic-specific prior knowledge that reflects information that is either not explicitly in the text or cannot be inferred from the existing text information (Paul, 2001, 2003). It appears that many readers who are deaf or hard of hearing do not have adequate prior knowledge, do not apply it during reading, or do not have the opportunities to use or develop this skill. So far, there is no comprehensive model to understand the role of prior knowledge and reading comprehension for readers who are deaf or hard of hearing (Paul, 2003).

Wilson's (1979) study investigated the abilities of both students who are deaf or hard of hearing and hearing peers to answer text-explicit and inferential questions. Both groups of students showed difficulties in answering inferential questions. Jackson and colleagues (Jackson, Paul, & Smith, 1997) were interested in the contribution of prior knowledge to the students' ability to answer text-explicit and two levels of inferential questions. The 51 participants were 12- to 20-year-old adolescents who were deaf or hard of hearing. Results showed that participants' recall of information was positively promoted by detailed and additional probes in the pretest.

A few studies have attempted to explore whether particular strategies could assist the activation of students' prior knowledge. For example, the study conducted by Andrews and colleagues (Andrews, Winograd, & DeVille, 1994) found that the retelling performance of readers who used American Sign Language (ASL) summaries before reading exceeded their performance on stories without ASL summaries and exceeded the performance of the hearing readers who received no summary treatment. Al-Hilawani (2003) noted that the *key word* strategy (in which the teacher discusses story content with students and teaches students to select key words and then discusses those words before reading) improved comprehension and vocabulary for elementary school–aged students. On the other hand, a study conducted by Schirmer and Winter (1993) found no support for the use of thematic organizers to sufficiently activate prior knowledge for readers who are deaf or hard of hearing to comprehend narrative text.

In sum, studies on prior knowledge with readers who are deaf or hard of hearing have confirmed the conclusion of Schirmer and McGough's (2005) meta-analysis that building and activating prior knowledge directly influences reading comprehension, although no instructional strategies show conclusive effectiveness.

Research on Metacognition of Students Who Are Deaf or Hard of Hearing

During the preschool years, **metalingustic** insights about the language domains (e.g. phonology, morphology, syntax, semantics, and pragmatics) emerge and continue to develop throughout childhood and adolescence. Metalingustically, children can use language for thought and for communication, which involves the ability to play with the language, talk about it, analyze it, and make judgments about acceptable versus incorrect forms. Metacognition is a critical area, and its absence is noticeable in children who have language difficulties or who have not developed a high level of skill in the use of their language (Paul, 2001).

Because metacognition is related to so many different areas of reading comprehension, the research on metacognition with readers who are deaf or hard of hearing has proceeded in several directions. One line of research has been focused on readers' knowledge of text structure through retelling. Griffith and Ripich (1988) were interested in evaluating whether the retellings of readers who are deaf or hard of hearing were consistent with story structure elements. The 11 participants were 6- to 15-year-old students who are deaf or hard of hearing in a total communication program. The results confirmed the ability of students who are deaf or hard of hearing to use story structure in organizing their retellings. By assessing students' retelling performance, Donin, Doehring, and Browns (1991) investigated whether any particular structure supported significantly better comprehension than others; however, the findings did not support this hypothesis. In a case study conducted by Luetke-Stahlman and colleagues (Luetke-Stahlman, Griffiths, & Montgomery, 1998), a 7-year-old deaf child produced longer retellings with increasing targeted story structure components when the teacher emphasized the targeted text structures during the 28-week intervention period. Another line of research on readers' knowledge of text structure has been assessed by the students' written product (Akamatsu, 1988; Cambra, 1994; Schirmer, 1993; Schirmer & Bond, 1990).

A study conduced by Pakulski and Kaderavek (2001) not only confirmed the narrative ability (story retelling) of readers who are deaf or hard of hearing, but also suggested the effectiveness of role playing in improving readers' retelling skills. The participants were 14 students who were deaf or hard of hearing and who communicated orally. After repeated readings of two stories and role playing of one story, the participants' narrative products were evaluated. The findings indicated that the participants were able to accomplish the story retelling task and that the sophistication and complexity of their retelling improved with role playing.

Research studies conducted with readers who are deaf or hard of hearing have been focused on assessing the students' comprehension-monitoring skills through various approaches. For example, Davey (1987) documented better comprehension with the look-back technique for both readers who are deaf or hard or hearing and hearing, but the results also indicated that readers who are deaf or hard of hearing were not aware of their better performance using the look-back technique. Other studies have attempted to assess readers' comprehension-monitoring skills using direct approaches such as think-aloud or interviews. For example, comparing the comprehension-monitoring strategies of readers who are deaf or hard of hearing to those of hearing peers, Andrews and Mason (1991) asked the participants to think aloud when filling in the blank words or phrases in passages. Similar strategies were found to be used by both groups, although the strategies used by participants who are deaf or hard of hearing differed from those of the hearing participants by frequency and type. Both Ewoldt (1986) and Strassman (1992) interviewed students who are deaf or hard of hearing to investigate their comprehension-monitoring strategies directly and found that they did not use these strategies extensively.

In sum, a strong positive relationship between metacognitive skill and reading comprehension ability has been supported by research with both readers who are deaf or hard of hearing and hearing readers. However, compared to their hearing peers, readers who are deaf or hard of hearing generally demonstrate less metacognitive awareness. The research on metacognition skills of readers who are deaf or hard of hearing has been mostly assessment studies, so there is a significant need for more instructional efforts in this area.

How Comprehension Instruction Is Different for Students Who Are Deaf or Hard of Hearing

As previously discussed, vocabulary knowledge and reading comprehension are strongly related. Vocabulary knowledge supports overall understanding of text and that understanding then facilitates the learning of new words. The fact that children who are deaf or hard of hearing know fewer English words clearly influences their comprehension process, but this does not completely explain the comprehension difficulties they experience when reading. Syntactic and other language-related competence in English is also a factor (Wang, Kretschmer, & Hartman, 2008). Using the small amount of research available with readers who are deaf and hard of hearing and the underlying assumption that reading requires an awareness of the structure of language, it might be suggested that syntactic and other language-related strategies must be emphasized with readers who are deaf and hard of hearing—for example, figurative language, prior knowledge, and metacognition.

Meanwhile, in a comprehensive review on *Effects of Cochlear Implants on Children's Reading and Academic Achievement* (Marschark, Rhoten, & Fabich, 2007), the authors concluded that although the English language competence made possible by cochlear implantation has been shown to improve literacy skills of students who are deaf or hard of hearing (for example, see Vermeulen, van Bon, Schreuder, Knoors, & Snik, 2007), the empirical results are not always consistent. That is, cochlear implantation alone cannot guarantee better reading comprehension.

In addition to the recommendations of the National Reading Panel (2000), Luckner and his colleagues (Luckner, Sebald, Cooney, Young, & Goodwin Muir, 2005/2006) recommend that readers who are deaf or hard of hearing need instruction in the grammatical principles of ASL or the use of ASL signs in some form of signed English and how to translate those signs into written English. Similarly, in her study titled *What Really Matters in the Early Literacy Development of Deaf Children*, Mayer (2007) suggested:

> There are two areas, fundamental to success in learning to read and write, that need to be given more explicit attention as we design and research early literacy programs for deaf children. These are (a) developing a foundation in the spoken and/or signed mode of the language to be written (i.e., English) and (b) focusing on those strategies that allow children to make the most effective connections between face-to-face language and text. (p. 425)

Promisingly, Gentry, Chinn, and Moulton's (2004/2005) study—which showed increased understanding of concepts presented in stories on CD-ROM when the presentations included ASL demonstrations that could be associated with the print and pictures—supports the need for instruction in making the link between ASL and other signed language and the text.

In fact, based on research of teaching reading to language-minority children, the *Committee on the Prevention of Reading Difficulties in Young Children* (Snow et al., 1998) suggested that:

> [i]t is clear that initial reading instruction in the first language does no harm, and it seems likely both from research findings and from theories about literacy development that initial reading instruction in the second language can have negative consequences for immediate and long-term achievement. This conclusion leads us to urge initial literacy

instruction in a child's native language whenever possible and to suggest that literacy instruction should not be introduced in any language before some reasonable level of oral proficiency in that language has been attained. (p. 238)

Particularly, in content area reading, the link between a face-to-face language (spoken or signed mode) and the printed text should be emphasized. For example, with a heavy reliance on textbooks and paper-and-pencil assessments, conventional science instruction and assessment present an unnecessary obstacle for many students who are deaf or hard of hearing and cannot successfully access and utilize the information in print. It is possible that materials in face-to-face language (i.e., **performance literacy,** see Chapter 8) can be used or adopted to perform the same or similar functions (e.g., comprehension or metacognitive) as **script literacy** materials in all or most of these instructional activities (Paul & Wang, 2006a, 2006b). Students can obtain maximized meaningful cues that assist them in interpreting the content (e.g., science concepts and knowledge) being communicated through performance literacy. Furthermore, through the contextualized use of performance literacy in scientific inquiry where the students obtain a background for comprehension through their interactions with objects in their surroundings, students who are deaf or hard of hearing can develop and practice metacognitive thinking skills while enhancing their scientific conceptual understanding. Such a curricular integration of inquiry-based science instruction and performance literacy could be a promising practice for students who are deaf or hard of hearing, particularly for assisting them in accessing the general education curriculum (Wang & Paul, in press).

Collectively, our review of reading comprehension instruction for students who are deaf or hard of hearing concurs with the mainstream theory on comprehension instruction that effective comprehension instruction for students who are deaf or hard of hearing should be *balanced comprehension instruction*, which includes (1) explicit and direct instruction, specifically on syntax and figurative language of English; and (2) a supportive classroom context that provides plenty of time and opportunity for actual reading, writing, and discussion of the text for students to enrich their prior knowledge and to practice their metacognitive skills in particular. Above all, we strongly recommend the teaching of language-related reading comprehension strategies for students who are deaf or hard of hearing. We also highlight the link between performance literacy and script literacy in content area reading,

ASSESSMENTS OF COMPREHENSION

As stated in Chapters 4 through 6, an online database of reading assessments for students in kindergarten to second grade is available through the Southwest Educational Development Laboratory [SEDL] (2007). For this chapter, a search of tests assessing reading comprehension was conducted. This search yielded several norm- and criterion-referenced assessments. The names of the assessments, copyright, publisher, and Web site for each are summarized in Tables 7-1 and 7-2. As previously discussed, assessments such as these can assist teachers in understanding students' present level of performance and in developing appropriate annual goals and objectives in the area of reading comprehension. As discussed in Chapters 4 through 6, it is important for test administrators to review each subtest carefully to determine the effects of various administrative procedures to ensure that valid results are obtained.

TABLE 7-1 Norm-Referenced Assessments of Reading Comprehension

Name of Assessment	Copyright	Publisher	Web Site
Gates-MacGinitie Reading Tests, 4th edition (GMRT-4)	2002	Riverside Publishing Company	http://www.riverpub.com/
Gray Diagnostic Reading Tests, 2nd edition (GDRT-2)	2004	ProEd Publishing	http://www.proedinc.com/
Gray Oral Reading Test, 4th edition (GORT-4)	2001	Pearson Assessments	http://ags.pearsonassessments.com
Group Reading Assessment and Diagnostic Evaluation (GRADE)	2001	American Guidance Service, Inc.	http://www.agsnet.com/
Metropolitan Achievement Tests Reading Diagnostic Tests, 8th edition (MAT-8)	2002	The Psychological Corporation	http://psychcorp.com/
Qualitative Reading Inventory, 4th edition (QRI-4)	2006	Pearson/Allyn & Bacon	http://www.ablongman.com/
Standardized Reading Inventory, 2nd edition (SRI-2)	1999	ProEd Publishing	http://www.proedinc.com/
Stanford Achievement Test 10th Edition (SAT-10)	2004	Harcourt Assessment	http://www.harcourtassessment.com/
Test of Kindergarten/First Grade Readiness Skills	1987	Psychological and Educational Publications, Inc.	http://www.psych-edpublications.com/
Test of Oral Reading and Comprehension Skills (TORCS)	2000	Academic Therapy Publications	http://www.academictherapy.com/
Test of Reading Comprehension, 3rd edition (TORC-3)	1995	ProEd Publishing	http://www.proedinc.com/
Wechsler Individual Achievement Test, 2nd edition (WIAT-II)	2005	The Psychological Corporation	http://www.psychcorp.com/

INSTRUCTIONAL GOALS AND OBJECTIVES

As discussed in Chapters 4 through 6, writing instructional goals and objectives for Individualized Education Programs is an important first step in planning instructional interventions for students. On a yearly basis, teachers are required to write a present level of performance for each area of instructional need. This present level of performance summarizes results of formal and informal assessments and observational data pertaining to the student's classroom performance. After reviewing the information included in the present level of performance, the teacher must compose a measurable, instructional goal that describes what gain can be reasonably achieved given one year of instruction. Once the goal has been determined, benchmarks or short-term objectives are crafted to divide the annual goal into discrete, instructional

TABLE 7-2 Criterion-Referenced Assessments of Comprehension

Name of Assessment	Copyright	Publisher	Web Site
Analytical Reading Inventory, 7th edition	2003	Pearson Education	http://www.prenhall.com/
Bader Reading and Language Inventory, 5th edition	2005	Pearson Education	http://www.prenhall.com/
Developmental Reading Assessment, K-3, 2nd edition (DRA-2, K-3)	2006	Celebration Press Pearson Learning Group	http://www.pearsonlearning.com/
Dynamic Indicators of Basic Early Literacy Skills, 6th edition (DIBELS-6)	2007	University of Oregon	http://dibels.uoregon.edu/
Ekwall/Shanker Reading Inventory, 4th edition (ESRI-4)	2000	Pearson/Allyn & Bacon	http://www.ablongman.com/
Phonological Awareness Literacy Screening (PALS)	2005	University of Virginia	http://pals.virginia.edu
Reading Inventory for the Classroom, 5th edition (RIC)	2004	Pearson Education	http://www.prenhall.com/
Stieglitz Informal Reading Inventory, 3rd edition	2002	Pearson/Allyn & Bacon	http://www.ablongman.com/
Texas Primary Reading Inventory	2005	Texas Education Agency	http://www.txreadinginstruments.com/
The Critical Reading Inventory	2004	Pearson Education	http://www.prenhall.com/

components. A sample annual goal and short-term objectives to address a need in the area of reading comprehension is included in Table 7-3. This sample instructional goal was written to address the reading comprehension needs of Danielle, the student who is the subject of Case Study D. For further information regarding Danielle, please refer to the information provided in the case study section of the text.

COMPREHENSION INSTRUCTION

As with vocabulary instruction in Chapter 6, the *Consumer's Guide to Evaluating a Core Reading Program, Grades K–3: A Critical Elements Analysis* (Simmons & Kame'enui, 2003) recommended by the American Federation of Teachers [AFT] and utilized by the Oregon Reading First Center (2004) did not identify comprehension instruction as a critical element for instruction for students in kindergarten through third grade. However, as with Chapter 6, a *Review of Supplemental and Intervention Reading Programs* was compiled by Oregon Reading First Center. This report represents a review of hundreds of curricular programs focused on the development of beginning reading skills and is available online. In this chapter focusing on reading comprehension, the item analysis data for comprehension for each curriculum reviewed is available at http://oregonreadingfirst.uoregon.edu. In addition to the suggestions from the Oregon

TABLE 7-3 Annual Goal and Short-Term Objectives for Reading Comprehension

Area of Need: Reading Comprehension

Present Level of Performance:

Danielle uses American Sign Language (ASL) as her primary mode of communication and to acquire content knowledge in the classroom. Several subtests of the Woodcock-Johnson Test of Achievement-III were recently administered, and results indicate that Danielle's abilities in the areas of reading are below the standard score average of 100. Specifically, her score on the Letter–Word Identification subtest was 92, Word Attack 75, and Passage Comprehension 84. Results of an informal reading inventory suggest that Danielle's independent reading level is approximately at the third-grade level. These findings are consistent with her performance in the classroom. Although she can provide the correct signs for individual words as she reads, Danielle experiences difficulty understanding English syntax and answering comprehension questions about what was read and does not appear to monitor her comprehension as she reads. Danielle's interest and motivation for reading have recently increased, and her parents report that she is requesting to go to the library and wants a subscription to a teen magazine for her birthday.

Goal:

Given a selected passage written at her independent reading level, Danielle will apply the comprehension strategies she has learned to correctly answer 8 out of 10 written comprehension questions.

How will progress toward this goal be measured?

Comprehension quizzes and tests, teacher observation, review of assignments, student and parent reports.

Short-Term Objectives or Benchmarks Including Criteria for Evaluation

- Given instruction in comprehension-monitoring strategies (e.g., summarizing and questioning), Danielle will independently apply these strategies to read and comprehend materials written at her level and report successful attempts of using these strategies to her teacher and parents.

- When asked to sequence the events of a story or summarize the main events of a selection read independently, Danielle will use a graphic organizer in 8 out of 10 instances to organize her thoughts before writing.

- Using her previously created and reviewed graphic organizer, Danielle will transfer the information into at least one written paragraph containing an introductory sentence, three supporting details, and a conclusion sentence.

- Danielle will seek assistance from an adult only after she has attempted at least one newly acquired comprehension strategy.

- Given instruction in English syntax, Danielle will practice translating concepts and phrases presented in ASL into English sentences and ask an adult to review them in 8 out of 10 instances.

Progress Toward Annual Goal

Date	Progress*	Comments:

*Minimal (M): anticipate that the goal will not be met by the end of the quarter
Proficient (P): anticipate that the goal will be met by the end of the quarter
Advanced (A): anticipate that the goal will be exceeded by the end of the quarter

Reading First Center, the AFT also recommends that teachers explore the What Works Clearinghouse (http://ies.ed.gov/ncee/wwc/) and the Florida Center for Reading Research (http://www.fcrr.org) for information regarding effective reading comprehension interventions and instructional strategies.

As mentioned in Chapters 4 through 6, we encourage readers to explore the resources provided above to identify successful reading comprehension interventions to implement with students who are deaf or hard of hearing. In addition to published reading curriculums, many print and online resources are available to provide teachers with ideas for implementing effective reading comprehension instruction in the classroom. A list of these teacher resources is included at the end of this chapter. In addition, teacher-created materials may also be used to address reading comprehension instruction. A description of several activities is provided in the following section.

Comprehension Instructional Activities

The National Reading Panel (2000) identified six research-based instructional strategies to promote improved reading comprehension skills among students: (1) comprehension monitoring, (2) using graphic and semantic organizers, (3) answering questions, (4) generating questions, (5) recognizing story structure, and (6) summarizing. Furthermore, the panel suggested that effective comprehension strategy instruction (1) is explicit or direct, (2) can be accomplished through cooperative

learning, and (3) helps readers use comprehension strategies flexibly and in combination with one another. In accordance with these recommendations, the following instructional activities are presented.

- *Story Pyramid:* Using the graphic organizer illustrated in Figure 7-1, students complete each line of the pyramid with a different piece of information from the text. The questions can vary depending on the type of selection the students are reading (e.g., fiction versus nonfiction). Graphic organizers can be utilized to promote comprehension monitoring, answering and generating questions, recognizing story structure, and summarizing; therefore, they are an excellent example of using comprehension strategies in conjunction with one another. In addition, teachers can use graphic organizers to support their direct instruction of comprehension strategies as well as guide students through cooperative learning activities. Houghton

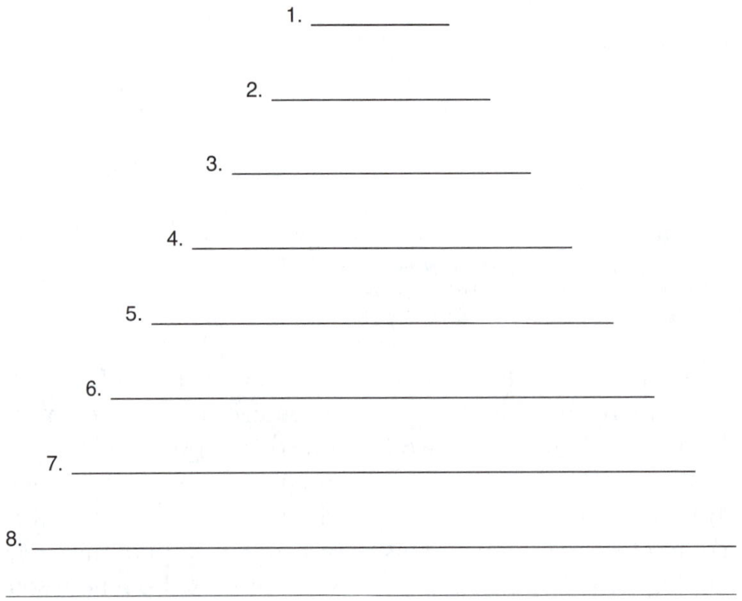

1. _____

2. _____

3. _____

4. _____

5. _____

6. _____

7. _____

8. _____

_____

FIGURE 7-1 *Story Pyramid*

Mifflin's *Education Place* Web site (http://www.eduplace.com/graphicorganizer/) provides a variety of graphic organizers for different purposes.

1. Write the name of the main character.

2. Write two words that describe the main character.

3. Write three words that describe the setting of the story.

4. Write four words that state the problem of the story.

5. Write five words that describe the first major event that occurred in the story.

6. Write six words that describe the second major event that occurred in the story.

7. Write seven words that describe the third major event that occurred in the story.

8. Write eight words that describe the outcome of the story.

- *Comic Strip:* This activity can be completed individually, with partners, or in a cooperative group. After reading a selection, the teacher directs the students to fold a piece of white paper into fourths, sixths, or eighths, depending on the number of events in the reading selection. Students then create a comic strip that illustrates and summarizes the main events that occurred in the selection in the proper sequence.

- *Post-it!* Post-it notes provide an excellent way for students to monitor their comprehension while reading. In this activity, the teacher provides students with a package of small Post-it notes and directs them to focus on a particular comprehension strategy such as generating questions. As students read through the selection, they note a question on the Post-it and place it directly in the text where they would ask the question. For example, a student may generate a simple question such as "What is the main character's name?" or a higher-level question such as "What motivated Brandon to contact the authorities at this point in the story? Provide evidence from earlier in the chapter to support your viewpoint." Similarly, larger Post-it notes can be used when writing short summaries about a selection read. As with the generating questions activity, students can place the larger Post-it note directly in the text to indicate a summation of a particular section.

- *Sketch to Stretch:* This activity encourages nonverbal responses for comprehension and allows students to "stretch" their thinking about what they are reading. As students are reading a selection, the teacher stops them periodically and provides them with one minute to construct a sketch. The sketch does not have to be an artistic rendition of what is being read but something that symbolizes a main idea, thought, question, or other connection to the text. After reading, students can be divided into groups to discuss their drawings and offer interpretations of each other's sketches.

ADDITIONAL CONSIDERATIONS ASSOCIATED WITH READING COMPREHENSION INSTRUCTION

According to the National Reading Panel (2000), teachers' questions support and advance the reading comprehension abilities of students. Teachers' questions provide a purpose for reading, focus attention on what to learn, encourage active thinking, assist in comprehension monitoring, and allow students to review content. In addition, the types of questions posed and modeled by the teacher strongly influence the questions students will generate for themselves. For many students, including those who are deaf or hard of hearing, prior knowledge also plays a key role in reading comprehension abilities. As authors of this text, we believe that it is crucial that teachers of the deaf and hard of hearing focus additional attention on question types and building prior knowledge. Therefore, an overview of the **Taxonomy of Educational Objectives,** often called **Bloom's Taxonomy** (Bloom, 1956), and the Core Knowledge Curriculum is provided in the following sections.

Bloom's Taxonomy

Bloom's Taxonomy was first proposed in 1956 by Benjamin Bloom, an educational psychologist at the University of Chicago. Bloom's Taxonomy divides objectives and skills for student learning into three domains: affective, psychomotor, and cognitive. The original goal of Bloom's Taxonomy was to encourage educators to focus skill development in all three domains, thereby creating an increasingly holistic form of education. Like Chall's (1996) Stages of Reading Development, Bloom's Taxonomy is hierarchical in nature, meaning that the acquisition of skills at the higher levels depends on prerequisite knowledge and mastery of lower-level skills.

Although Bloom's Taxonomy (Bloom, 1956) was intended to incorporate three domains of learning, most references to the taxonomy focus primarily on the cognitive domain. The skills in this domain tend to be the focus of traditional education, particularly the lower-level skills. Bloom's Taxonomy is usually depicted in a triangular shape, with the base of the triangle representing the most frequently occurring question types and the top of the triangle the least. Beginning at the base of the triangle and moving upward, the categories of question types include (1) *knowledge* questions that assess the student's ability to recall or remember basic facts, (2) *comprehension* questions that focus on the student's ability to explain ideas or concepts, (3) *application* questions that allow the teacher to judge the student's ability to use information in a new way, (4) *analysis* questions that evaluate the student's ability to distinguish between different segments of information, (5) *synthesis* questions that determine whether or not the student can justify a stand or position and (6) *evaluation* questions that are aimed at assessing whether or not the student can create a new product or point of view.

In the 1990s, a former student of Bloom's led a group in updating and revising the taxonomy. The resulting revised version of the taxonomy (Anderson & Krathwohl, 2001) used verbs rather than nouns to represent the different hierarchical levels. Consequently, the six levels of question types from the bottom to the top of the Bloom Taxonomy are (1) remembering, (2) understanding, (3) applying, (4) analyzing, (5) evaluating, and (6) creating (see details on both the old and new version of Bloom's Taxonomy at http://www.odu.edu). In addition to the changes proposed by Anderson and Krathwohl, other researchers have suggested that even though the three lowest levels appear to be hierarchically ordered, the three higher levels should be viewed as parallels. Regardless of the configuration or labels used, we suggest that teachers use Bloom's Taxonomy to assist them in formulating questions for students and encourage students to use the taxonomy to guide them in generating questions at various levels. Several resources containing sample questioning formats and ideas for incorporating Bloom's Taxonomy into classroom activities are provided at the end of this chapter.

Core Knowledge Curriculum

In a recent review of the basal reading series used with young readers, Walsh (2003) discussed the shortcomings of basal reading programs as related to the development of word- and domain-specific background knowledge necessary for increasing reading comprehension abilities. Referring to the work of Chall (1996), Walsh stated that "[i]n order to make the transition from 'learning to read' to 'reading to learn' described by Jeanne Chall, children must have a foundation of broad vocabulary and world knowledge that includes important domains and is built up over time" (p. 24). She further indicated that children from mid- to high-income homes acquire this prior knowledge at home, but that many children from low-income homes depend on teachers and the chosen reading series for the development of this knowledge.

Specifically, Walsh (2003) referred to the following three reasons why basal reading series fail to adequately address the development of background knowledge. She indicated that these series (1) do not focus on systematically building essential knowledge and vocabulary during teacher read-alouds and discussions aimed at building background knowledge; (2) include many more lessons on formal reading comprehension skills than researchers have found are needed; and (3) offer mostly incoherent, banal themes and miss opportunities to develop word and world knowledge by offering and exploiting content-rich themes. The conclusion reached by Schirmer and McGough (2005) is that building and activating prior knowledge directly influences reading comprehension for readers who are deaf or hard of hearing. This ensures that the chosen basal reading series adequately, systematically, and explicitly addresses the National Reading Panel's (2000) recommended instructional strategies, a goal of utmost importance.

The American Federation of Teachers (AFT) (2007) echoed Walsh's (2003) observations and reiterated the importance of building background knowledge and its relation to reading comprehension. The AFT suggested that a knowledge-rich curriculum is particularly critical for (1) children from low-income families, who, on average, "have been exposed to roughly 30 million fewer words than children from professional families" (p. 1); and (2) students whose word and world knowledge is less developed compared to their peers. Given the discussion of vocabulary and language delays in Chapter 6 and prior knowledge here in Chapter 7, it is clear that these statements apply to many students who are deaf or hard of hearing.

To begin to alleviate this issue and ensure that all children, regardless of background, are exposed to rich, broad knowledge, the AFT (2007) recommended the use of a common core curriculum and specifically highlighted the Core Knowledge Curriculum developed by E. D. Hirsch, who founded the Core Knowledge Foundation in 1987 and published *The Schools We Need and Why We Don't Have Them* in 1996. Since 1997, Hirsch has begun writing the books that now make up the Core Knowledge series. The series contains seven books describing the content knowledge that should be taught at each grade level from kindergarten through sixth grade. Currently, there are schools in nearly all 50 states that have adopted the Core Knowledge series as their primary curriculum. As with many of the other curricular interventions reviewed in this book, we suggested that educators working with children and adolescents who are deaf or hard of hearing explore the Core Knowledge series and evaluate its effectiveness for developing prior knowledge for these students.

Conclusion

This chapter focused on reading comprehension instruction for children and adolescents who are deaf or hard of hearing. The recommendations of the National Reading Panel (2000) and a synthesis of the available research on deaf or hard of hearing individuals were the primary sources used to guide this discussion. Reading comprehension refers to the ability to obtain meaning from written text for some purpose. The primary components of proficient comprehension are adequate word recognition and advanced development of language comprehension and knowledge-acquisition skills. Effective comprehension instruction for students who are deaf or hard of hearing should be *balanced comprehension instruction* that emphasizes explicit and direct instruction, particularly on syntax and figurative language of English, as well as building a supportive classroom environment that provides plenty of time and opportunity for actual reading, writing, and discussion of the text for students to enrich their prior knowledge and practice their metacognitive skills. The teaching of language-related reading comprehension strategies for students who are deaf or hard of hearing is strongly suggested.

Chapter Summary

- According to the National Reading Panel (2000), six recommended strategies appear to have a solid scientific basis for enhancing text comprehension: (1) comprehension monitoring, (2) using graphic and semantic organizers, (3) answering questions, (4) generating questions, (5) recognizing story structure, and (6) summarizing. Effective comprehension strategy instruction (1) is explicit or direct, (2) can be accomplished through cooperative learning, and (3) helps readers use comprehension strategies flexibly and in combination with one another. Making use of prior knowledge and using mental imagery are two additional reading comprehension strategies that have received some scientific support.

- Because of the close relationship between reading comprehension and language comprehension and the language deficit of most deaf students and many students who are hard of hearing, it is not difficult to understand the lower levels of reading comprehension compared to hearing peers. The majority of research conducted on the reading comprehension abilities of students who are deaf or hard of hearing focuses on four main areas: (1) syntactic knowledge, (2) figurative language, (3) prior knowledge, and (4) metacognition.

- Bloom's Taxonomy is a model that divides objectives and skills for student learning into three domains: affective, psychomotor, and cognitive. It is hierarchical in nature—that is, the acquisition of skills at the higher levels depends on prerequisite knowledge and mastery of lower level skills. Teachers are encouraged to use this hierarchical model to develop comprehension questions for students. Furthermore, teachers should provide instruction in using the taxonomy to guide students in generating questions.

- There is also a need for a common core curriculum for developing students' prior knowledge.

REVIEW QUESTIONS

1. The National Reading Panel (2000) recommended six instructional strategies for developing reading comprehension skills. What are the six strategies, and how would you describe them?

2. What are the three recommended instructional arrangements for teaching reading comprehension strategies?

3. What are the major findings and conclusions of the research conducted on the reading comprehension abilities of students who are deaf or hard of hearing in the following four areas: (1) syntactic knowledge, (2) figurative language, (3) prior knowledge and (4) metacognition?

REFLECTIVE QUESTIONS

1. How would you describe the difficulties that students who are deaf or hard of hearing experience with reading comprehension to a teacher in the general education environment?

2. What strategies would you use to improve a student's prior knowledge on a particular topic prior to reading a selection? Provide a brief description of the topic and several examples of the strategies you would employ.

APPLICATION EXERCISES

1. Using the annual goal and objective presented in this chapter, write a week-long lesson plan to address one of the short-term objectives written for Danielle.

2. Write a present level of performance, an annual goal, and at least three short-term objectives to address the reading comprehension needs of Carlos, the subject of Case Study C.

3. Using a short reading selection or a chapter from a book, create a list of questions that utilize all six level of Bloom's Taxonomy for that selection and label your questions accordingly.

SUGGESTED READINGS AND RESOURCES

Readings

Bray, P. P., & Rogers, J. M. (2002). *Ideas in Bloom: Taxonomy-based activities for U.S. studies, Grades 7–9.* Portland, ME: Walch Publishing.

Brown, L. (2005). *How to make your classroom Bloom: Success on standardized tests using Bloom's taxonomy.* Mooresville, NC: Performance Education.

Feeney Honson, K. (2005). *Sixty strategies for improving reading comprehension in grades K–8*. Thousand Oaks, CA: Corwin Press.

Graff Silver, R. (2003). *First graphic organizers: Reading; 30 reproducible graphic organizers that build early reading and comprehension skills*. New York: Scholastic.

Hirsch, E. D. & Holdren, J. (Eds.) (1996). *Books to build on: A grade-by-grade resource guide for parents and teachers (Core Knowledge series)*. New York: Dell.

Irwin-DeVitis, L., Bromley, K., & Modlo, M. (1999). *Fifty graphic organizers for reading, writing and more (grades 4–8)*. New York: Scholastic.

Klingner, J. K., Vaughn, S. & Boardman, A. (2007). *Teaching reading comprehension to students with learning difficulties (what works for special-needs learners)*. New York: Guilford Press.

Pinnell, G. S. & Scharer, P. (2003). *Teaching for comprehension in reading, grades K–2*. New York: Scholastic.

Resources

Bloom's taxonomy
   http://www.teachers.ash.org.au/
   researchskills/dalton.htm
   http://www.nwlink.com/~donclark/hrd/
   bloom.html

Comprehension instruction
   http://www.tengrrl.com/tens/016.shtml
   http://web2.uvcs.uvic.ca/elc/studyzone/
   http://www.resourceroom.net/
   Comprehension/index.asp
   http://members.tripod.com/%7Eemu1967/
   readstrat.htm

Graphic organizers
   http://edhelper.com/teachers/graphic_
   organizers.htm
   http://www.region15.org/curriculum/
   graphicorg.html
   http://www.graphicorganizers.com/

REFERENCES

Akamatsu, C. T. (1988). Summarizing stories: The role of instruction in text structure in learning to write. *American Annals of the Deaf, 133*, 294–302.

Al-Hilawani, Y. A. (2003). Clinical examination of three methods of teaching reading comprehension to deaf and hard-of-hearing students: From research to classroom applications. *Journal of Deaf Studies and Deaf Education,8* (2), 145–156.

American Federation of Teachers. (2007). Common, knowledge-rich curriculum. *Charting the Course*. Washington, DC: Author.

Anderson, L.W., & Krathwohl, D. R. (Eds.). (2001). *A taxonomy for learning, teaching, and assessing: A revision of Bloom's Taxonomy of educational objectives*. New York: Longman.

Andrews, J. F., & Mason, J. (1991). Strategies use among deaf and hearing readers. *Exceptional Children, 57*, 536–545.

Andrews, J. F., Winograd, P., & DeVille, G. (1994). Deaf children reading fables: Using ASL summaries to improve reading comprehension. *American Annals of the Deaf, 139*, 378–386.

Armbruster, B. B., Lehr, F., & Osborn, J. (2001). *Put reading first: The research building blocks for teaching children to read kindergarten through grade three.* Jessup, MD: National Institute for Literacy.

Bernhardt, E. (1991). *Reading development in a second language.* Norwood, NJ: Ablex.

Bloom, B. S. (1956). *Taxonomy of educational objectives, handbook 1: The cognitive domain.* White Plains, NY: Longman-New York.

Cambra, C. (1994). An instructional program approach to improve hearing-impaired adolescents' narratives: A pilot study. *Volta Review, 96,* 237–245.

Chall, J. S. (1996). *Stages of reading development.* (2nd ed.). New York: McGraw-Hill.

Chomsky, N. (1957). *Syntactic structures.* The Hague, Netherlands: Mouton.

Chomsky, N. (1965). *Aspects of the theory of syntax.* Cambridge: MIT Press.

Chomsky, N. (1975). *Reflections on language.* New York: Pantheon Books.

Chomsky, N. (1988). *Language and problems of knowledge: The Managua lectures.* Cambridge: MIT Press.

Conley, J. (1976). Role of idiomatic expressions in the reading of deaf children. *American Annals of the Deaf, 121,* 381–385.

Davey, B. (1987). Postpassage questions: Task and reader effects on comprehension and metacomprehension processes. *Journal of Reading Behavior, 19,* 261–283.

Diebold, T. J., & Waldron, M. B. (1988). Designing instructional formats: The effects of verbal and pictorial components on hearing-impaired students' comprehension of science concepts. *American Annals of the Deaf, 133,* 3–35.

Donin, J., Doehring, D. G., & Browns, F. (1991). Text comprehension and reading achievement in orally educated hearing-impaired children. *Discourse Processes, 14,* 307–337.

Duke, N. K., & Pearson, P. D. (2003). Effective practices for developing reading comprehension. In A. E. Farstrup & S. J. Samuels (Eds.), *What research has to say about reading instruction* (3rd ed.) (pp. 205–242). Newark, DE: International Reading Association.

Durkin, D. (1978). What classroom observations reveal about reading comprehension instruction. *Reading Research Quarterly, 14,* 481–533.

Ewoldt, C. (1981). A psycholinguistic description of selected deaf children reading in sign language. *Reading Research Quarterly, 17,* 58–89.

Ewoldt, C. (1986). What does "reading" mean? *Perspectives for Teachers of the Hearing Impaired, 4,* 10–13.

Fruchter, A., Wilbur, R., & Fraser, B. (1984). Comprehension of idioms by hearing-impaired students. *Volta Reviews, 86,* 7–18.

Gentry, M. M., Chinn, K. M., & Moulton, R. D. (2004/2005). Effectiveness of multimedia reading materials when used with children who are deaf. *American Annals of the Deaf, 149* (5), 394–403.

Griffith, P. L., & Ripich, D. N. (1988). Story structure recall in hearing-impaired, learning-disabled, and nondisabled children. *American Annals of the Deaf, 133,* 43–50.

Hirsch, E. D. (1996). *The schools we need and why we don't have them.* New York: Doubleday.

Iran-Nejad, A., Ortony, A., & Rittenhouse, R. (1981). The comprehension of metaphorical uses of English by deaf children.

Journal of Speech and Hearing Research, 24, 551–556.

Israelite, N. K., & Helfrich, M. A. (1988). Improving text coherence in basal readers: Effects of revisions on the comprehension of hearing-impaired and normal hearing readers. *Volta Review, 90,* 261–176.

Jackson, D. W., Paul, P. V., & Smith, J. C. (1997). Prior knowledge and reading comprehension ability of deaf adolescents. *Journal of Deaf Studies and Deaf Education, 2,* 172–184.

Kelly, L. (1998). Using silent motion pictures to teach complex syntax to adult deaf readers. *Journal of Deaf Studies and Deaf Education, 3,* 217–230.

King, C., & Quigley, S. (1985). *Reading and deafness.* San Diego: College Hill Press.

Lillo-Martin, D., Hanson, V., & Smith, S. (1991). Deaf readers' comprehension of complex syntactic structure. In D. Martin (Ed.), *Advances in cognition, education, and deafness* (pp. 146–151). Washington, DC: Gallaudet University Press.

Lillo-Martin, D., Hanson, V., & Smith, S. (1992). Deaf readers' comprehension of relative clause structure. *Applied Psycholinguistics, 13,* 13–30.

Luckner, J. L., Sebald, A. N., Cooney, J., Young, J., & Goodwin Muir, S. (2005/2006). An examination of the evidence-based literacy research in deaf education. *American Annals of the Deaf, 150* (5), 443–456.

Luetke-Stahlman, B., Griffiths, C., & Montgomery, N. (1998). Development of text structure knowledge as assessed by spoken and signed retellings of a deaf second-grade student. *American Annals of the Deaf, 143,* 337–346.

Marschark, M., Rhoten, C., & Fabich, M. (2007). Effects of cochlear implants on children's reading and academic achievement. *Journal of Deaf Studies and Deaf Education, 12,* 269–282.

Mayer, C. (2007). What really matters in the early literacy development of deaf children. *Journal of Deaf Studies and Deaf Education, 12,* 411–431.

McGill-Franzen, A., & Gormley, K. (1980). The influence of context on deaf readers' understanding of passive sentences. *American Annals of the Deaf, 125,* 937–942.

McGuinness, D. (2004). *Early reading instruction: What science really tells us about how to teach reading.* Cambridge: MIT Press.

McGuinness, D. (2005). Language development and learning to read: The scientific study of how language development affects reading skill. Cambridge: MIT Press.

McKnight, T. K. (1989). The use of cumulative cloze to investigate contextual build-up in deaf and hearing readers. *American Annals of the Deaf, 134,* 268–272.

Miller, P. F. (2000). Syntactic and semantic processing in Hebrew readers with prelingual deafness. *American Annuals of the Deaf, 145,* 436–451.

Miller, P. (2005) Reading comprehension and its relation to the quality of functional hearing: Evidence from readers with different functional hearing abilities. *American Annals of the Deaf, 150* (3), 305–323.

National Reading Panel. (2000). *Report of the National Reading Panel: Teaching children to read—An evidence-based assessment of the scientific research literature on reading and its implications for reading instruction.* Jessup, MD: National Institute for Literacy at EDPubs.

Nolen, S., & Wilbur, R. (1985). The effects of context on deaf students' comprehension of difficult sentences. *American Annals of the Deaf, 130,* 231–235.

Oregon Reading First Center. (2004). *Review of comprehensive reading programs.* Retrieved October 21, 2007, from http://reading.uoregon.edu/curricula/intro_summ_review_3-04.pdf.

Orlando, A., & Shulman, B. (1989). Severe-to-profound hearing-impaired children's comprehension of figurative language. *Journal of Childhood Communication Disorders, 12,* 157–165.

Pakulski, L. A., & Kaderavek, J. N. (2001). Narrative production by children who are deaf or hard of hearing: The effect of role-play. *Volta Review, 103* (3), 127–139.

Paris, S., & Stahl, S. (Eds.). (2005). *Children's reading comprehension and assessment.* Mahwah, NJ: Erlbaum.

Paul, P. (1998). *Literacy and deafness: The development of reading, writing, and literate thought.* Needham Heights, MA: Allyn & Bacon.

Paul, P. (2001). *Language and deafness* (3rd ed.). San Diego: Singular Thomson Learning.

Paul, P. (2003). Processes and components of reading. In M. Marschark & P. Spencer (Eds.), *Handbook of deaf studies, language, and education* (97–109). New York: Oxford University Press.

Paul, P., & Wang, Y. (2006a). Literate thought and deafness: A call for a new perspective and line of research on literacy. *The Punjab University Journal of Special Education (Pakistan), 2* (1), 28–37.

Paul, P., & Wang, Y. (2006b). Literate thought and multiple literacies. *Theory into Practice, 45* (4), 304–310.

Payne, J-A., & Quigley, S. (1987). Hearing-impaired children's comprehension of verb-particle combinations. *Volta Review, 89,* 133–143.

Quigley, S., McAnally, P., King, C., & Rose, S. (1991). *Reading milestones.* Austin, TX: Pro-Ed.

Quigley, S., Power, D., & Steinkamp, M. (1977). The language structure of deaf children. *Volta Review, 79,* 73–83.

Quigley, S., Smith, N., & Wilbur, R. (1974). Comprehension of relativized sentences by deaf students. *Journal of Speech and Hearing Research, 17,* 325–341.

Quigley, S., Wilbur, R., & Montanelli, D. (1974). Question formation in the language of deaf students. *Journal of Speech and Hearing Research, 17,* 699–713.

Quigley, S., Wilbur, R., & Montanelli, D. (1976). Complement structures in the language of deaf students. *Journal of Speech and Hearing Research, 19,* 448–457.

Schirmer, B. R. (1993). Constructing meaning from narrative text: Cognitive processes of deaf children. *American Annals of the Deaf, 138,* 397–403.

Schirmer, B. R., & Bond, W. L. (1990). Enhancing the hearing impaired child's knowledge of story structure to improve comprehension of narrative text. *Reading Improvement, 27,* 242–254.

Schirmer, B. R., & McGough, S. M. (2005). Teaching reading to children who are deaf: Do the conclusions of the National Reading Panel apply? *Review of Educational Research, 75* (1), 83–117.

Schirmer, B. R., & Winter, C. R. (1993). Use of cognitive schema by children who are deaf for comprehending narrative text. *Reading Improvement, 30,* 26–34.

Simmons, D. C., & Kame'enui, E. J. (2003). *A consumer's guide to evaluating a core reading program, grades K-3: A critical elements analysis.* Retrieved October 21, 2007, from http://teacher.scholastic.com/products/fundingconnection/pdf/Kameenui_GR_Blue.pdf

Snow, C., Burns, S., & Griffin, P. (Eds.). (1998). *Preventing reading difficulties in young children.* Washington, DC: National Academy Press.

Snow, C. E., Griffin, P., & Burns, M. S. (Eds.). (2005). *Knowledge to support the teaching of reading: Preparing teachers for a changing world.* San Francisco, CA: John Wiley & Sons, Inc.

Southwest Educational Development Laboratory. (2007). *Reading assessment database.* Retrieved March 3, 2007, from http://www.sedl.org/reading/rad/database.html.

Stoefen-Fisher, J. M. (December 1987–January 1988). Hearing-impaired adolescents' comprehension of anaphoric relationship within conjoined sentences. *Journal of Special Education, 21,* 85–98.

Strassman, B. K. (1992). Deaf adolescents' metacognitive knowledge about school-related reading. *American Annals of the Deaf, 137,* 326–330.

Vellutino, F. R. (2003). Individual differences as sources of variability in reading comprehension in elementary school children. In A. P. Sweet & C. E. Snow (Eds.), *Rethinking reading comprehension* (pp. 51–81). New York: Guilford Press.

Vermeulen, A. M., van Bon, W., Schreuder, R., Knoors, H., & Snik, A. (2007). Reading comprehension of deaf children with cochlear implants. *Journal of Deaf Studies and Deaf Education, 12,* 283–302.

Walsh, K. (2003). Basal readers: The lost opportunity to build the knowledge that propels comprehension. *American Educator, Spring,* 24–27.

Wang, Y., Kretschmer, R. & Hartman, M. (2008). Reading and students who are d/Deaf or hard of hearing. *Journal of Balanced Reading Instruction, 15* (2), 53–68.

Wang, Y., & Paul, P. (in press). Inquiry-based science instruction and performance literacy for students with disabilities. *The Punjab University Journal of Special Education* (Pakistan).

Wilbur, R., Fraser, J., & Fruchter, A. (1981). *Comprehension of idioms by hearing-impaired students.* Paper presented at the American Speech-Language-Hearing Association Convention, Los Angeles.

Wilbur, R., & Goodhart, W. (1985). Comprehension of indefinite pronouns and quantifiers by hearing-impaired children. *Applied Psycholinguistics, 6,* 417–434.

Wilbur, R., Goodhart, W., & Fuller, D. (1989). Comprehension of English modals by hearing-impaired children. *Volta Review, 91,* 5–18.

Wilson, K. (1979). *Inference and language processing in hearing and deaf children.* Unpublished doctoral dissertation. Boston University, MA.

Yurkowski, P., & Ewoldt, C. (1986). A case for the semantic processing of the deaf reader. *American Annals of the Deaf, 131,* 243–247.

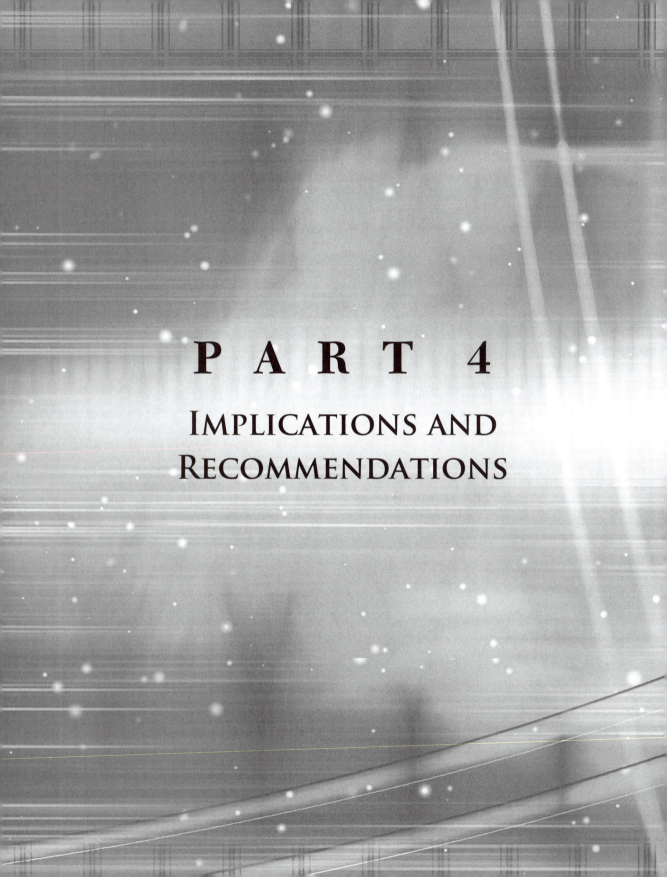

PART 4
IMPLICATIONS AND RECOMMENDATIONS

CHAPTER 8

READING AND LITERATE THOUGHT

All thinking involves perception, expectancies, inference, generalization, description, and judgment. Literate thought is the conscious representation and deliberate manipulation of those activities. Assumptions are universally made; literate thought is the recognition of an assumption as an assumption.... Even if literate thought is to a large extent ordinary thought rendered self-conscious and deliberate it is not tied exclusively to the practice of reading and writing. Literate thought can be, indeed is to some degree, embedded in the oral discourse of a literate society. We can talk of conjectures just as well as read and write about them. Literate thought is not restricted to the medium of writing even if writing and reading were critical in their evolution (Olson, 1994, pp. 280–281).

CHAPTER OBJECTIVES

After completing this chapter, the reader will be able to:

- Describe the major perspectives and findings on the concept of literate thought
- Explain the concepts of access and interpretation
- Discuss three types of literacies—script, caption, and performance
- Illustrate the implications for instructional practices for performance literacy including the use of process drama
- Describe the views on new and multiple literacies

INTRODUCTION

Thus far in this book, the focus has been on the development of reading skills in children and adolescents who are deaf or hard of hearing. We have attempted to apply the salient principles of Chall's (1996) model and other cognitive models (e.g., see discussions in Paul, 1998, 2003) and to incorporate the recommendations of the National Reading Panel (2000). There is little doubt that reading and writing are important skills, especially in a technologically driven society such as in the United States (Anderson, Hiebert, Scott, & Wilkinson, 1985; Snow, Burns, & Griffin, 1998). In other words, **literacy** (i.e., reading and writing) is critical for participating in and reaping the socioeconomic benefits of mainstream society. Obviously, literacy is essential for obtaining academic diplomas and degrees.

The passage at the head of this chapter (Olson, 1994) seems to imply that literacy is not really necessary for the development of **literate thought,** or even critical thinking, which—it can be argued—is one major or the major goal of education (e.g., Calfee, 1994; Paul, 1998, 2001; Paul & Wang, 2006a, 2006b). Literate thought has been defined as the ability to think in a creative, critical, complex, logical, rational, and reflective manner involving the use of literate language, which is often present or captured in printed materials such as books, journals, newspapers, and so on (Paul, 2006; Paul & Wang, 2006a, 2006b). However, according to Olson (1994), literate thought is possible via the use of and reflection on oral discourse, especially within a literate (print) society. Olson also asserts that literate thought involves the cognitive representation of information and manipulation of the contents of personal and social interactions and discussions. These views of Olson can also be gleaned from the various publications and discussions of the **new literacies and multiple literacies** that will be discussed later in this chapter (e.g., see discussions in Bloome & Paul, 2006; Paul, 2006).

Despite the importance of and focus on reading in this book, it is necessary to explore whether it is possible and feasible to develop literate thought in a mode other than print, especially for those children who have difficulty accessing or comprehending print materials. That is, is it possible to employ alternative means for presenting information that have been typically rendered primarily in print? The technology is already available for rendering such transliterated information in both oral forms (e.g., talking books, CDs) and sign forms (e.g., video books, DVDs).

Presenting information in these alternative modes is not sufficient for the development of literate thought. Then again, just because information is available in print and can be accessed by individuals does not necessarily mean that these individuals are literate thinkers. Regardless of how the information is captured (i.e., via print or nonprint modes), many children and adolescents need opportunities and possibly instruction and guidance to acquire higher-level skills such as comprehending, studying, remembering, synthesizing, and interpreting so that they can apply the captured information to other various situations (e.g., see discussions in Paris & Stahl, 2005;

Paul & Wang, 2006a, 2006b; Pearson & Fielding, 1991). In essence, individuals should become critical, literate thinkers regardless of the manner in which information is captured or accessed.

This chapter has several objectives. After providing some background on the concept of literate thought, we briefly describe three types of literacy—script, caption, and performance—that are relevant for individuals who are deaf or hard of hearing. To facilitate this discussion, it is necessary to provide a reconceptualization of the term literacy *and highlight the distinct and reciprocal relationship between* **access** *and* **interpretation**. *We then propose a few instructional implications involving the development of literate thought via performance literacy, including the use of* **process drama**. *Finally, the reader is introduced to the issues that have emerged because of the influence of new and multiple literacies. These new perspectives on literacy have called into question the predominant focus on print and on school literacy practices—that is, on the use of academic content materials and practices only in school settings.*

A Description of Literacy

Earlier in this book, we asked the question "What is reading?" and attempted to provide a historical perspective on the manner in which this term has been described. In this chapter, one of our major questions is "What is literacy?"; this is similar to the question "What is reading?" Traditionally and historically, literacy has been defined as the ability to read and write at some literate level (i.e., grade level) of society (e.g., Bartine, 1989, 1992). The answer to the question "What is literacy?" or "What is reading?" has been influenced by perspectives from an array of disciplines such as psychology, philosophy, sociology, literary criticism, and education (e.g., Bartine, 1989, 1992; Pearson, 2004; Pearson & Stephens, 1994). Even if we confine literacy to the domain of print (e.g., the alphabetic system of English), it should be clear that the authors of this book expect students who are deaf or hard of hearing to comprehend (access and understand) and interpret (use or apply in a critical manner) what they have read. Another way of saying this is that we expect these individuals to construct meaning that entails both the comprehension and interpretation processes.

It is critical to highlight two of these major concepts—*access* and *interpretation*—in order to understand our reconceptualized definition of literacy, which is discussed in greater detail later. With respect to English reading, we can describe access as the ability to decode the words in print that involves, among other factors, the need for fluent and accurate word-identification skills (see also the discussion on the *process-and-knowledge* view in Chapter 1). Interpretation entails understanding what one has read and then using that information during selected tasks such as making inferences within and across passages, stating your views on the topic, or critically evaluating the truthfulness of the information (e.g., Paris & Stahl, 2005; Pearson & Fielding, 1991; Pearson & Hamm, 2005). Interpretation depends on access skills. In fact, there is a reciprocal relation between access and interpretation, which is similar to the reciprocal relation between word identification and comprehension—as is the case for reading as discussed previously in this text.

Nevertheless, even if someone can access information, this does not necessarily mean that she can understand or interpret it. With respect to reading, we can safely say and—indeed have argued in the rest of this book—that one needs skills in, for example, the five National Reading Panel (2000) areas (phonemic awareness, text comprehension, etc.) to develop a good capacity in both the access and interpretation domains. The main goal of reading then is the comprehension and interpretation of print materials.

The discussion above illustrates what is now called *a narrow (or limited) perspective of literacy (or reading)*. That is, traditionally, literacy has been viewed as the ability to read and write via comprehension and interpretation or the construction of meaning (e.g., Bartine, 1989, 1992; Pearson & Hamm, 2005). From another perspective, literacy pertains to information presented via the mode of print—that is, the *world on paper* (Olson, 1994). For our purposes, the above views can be labeled as examples of script literacy.

We propose that literacy be reconceptualized as a form of *captured* literate information (e.g., Paul, 2006; Paul & Wang, 2006a, 2006b). Within this conceptual framework, English script literacy (i.e., print) is said to be captured (and represented) via the use of letters as part of the alphabetic system. **Literate information** refers to the style of information that has been presented in print materials—namely, abstract, complex, and removed from context, or, in other words, decontextualized information. This framework indicates that literate information can be captured also in nonprint modes such as audio books (via CDs) and video (i.e., signing) books (via DVDs). As is discussed later, we label these aforementioned nonprint modes as performance literacy.

This raises a couple of questions: Is it possible to develop literate thought via the use of nonprint modes? Would this approach be of the same quality as development in the script literacy mode? We do not wish to construe this as an either–or situation—that would be unproductive. First, we need to provide an example of our reconceptualized definition of literacy as a form of captured information through which we can adequately addressed these questions.

A Form of Captured Information

Consider the following passage, which contains a high-level use of literate language:

To think metaphysically is to think, without arbitrariness and dogmatism, on the most basic problems of existence. The problems are basic in the sense that they are fundamental, that much depends on them. Religion, for example, is not metaphysics; and yet if the metaphysical theory of materialism should be true, and it should thus be a fact that men have no souls, then much religion would founder on that fact. Again, moral philosophy is not metaphysics, and yet if the metaphysical theory of determinism should be true, or if the theory of fatalism should be true, many of our traditional presuppositions of morality would stand refuted by those truths. Similarly, logic is not metaphysics, and yet if it should turn out that, because of the nature of time, some assertions are neither true nor false, this would have serious implications for traditional logic. (Taylor, 1983, pp. 1–2)

With respect to the tasks of comprehension or interpretation, it should not matter whether an individual listens to or watches (in sign) a DVD version of the above passage (and thus, the entire book on metaphysics or reads the print version. Individuals should be able to replay the DVD (i.e., relisten or rewatch), jump ahead, stop it, and reflect about what they have heard or listened to, and so on. With advanced technology, one can maneuver back and forth with greater ease with the CD or DVD on the computer.

In a classroom situation, a teacher can ask specific questions about this passage (and the book) such as the following:

- What is the author's definition of metaphysics?
- Is religion or logic a form of metaphysics?
- What additional information would you need to understand what would be the downfall of religion or traditional logic?
- What questions do you have about this passage (book)?

These questions are similar to those which we would ask students if they were required to read the passage (or book). Is it easier to comprehend the information and answer the questions in print than in the nonprint CD or DVD mode? Why or why not? What would make this easier, especially since most people would agree that Taylor's *Metaphysics* is difficult to understand in any shape or form!

It is the *content* of captured information and the fact that it has been *captured* (preserved, recorded, etc.), whether in print or in some media format, that are important to consider. To develop literate thought, an individual needs not only to access the content in a particular form (print, audio book, etc.), but also to interpret and use this content. With guidance, support, and opportunity, similar to what we provide for print materials in classroom settings, children and adolescents who are deaf or hard of hearing as well other students, still should be able to develop a high level of literate thought because of their reflections on the captured form of information. Of course, these individuals may need to develop interpretation skills to accompany their access skills.

With the advent of technology, there are ample—almost endless—possibilities for developing literate thought for individuals who are deaf or hard of hearing. Even more important, especially for parents, this could be a viable way to help these individuals access the general education curriculum via alternative routes—that is, other than through the use of print materials. In the next section, the reader is introduced to some background for the concept of literate thought that will facilitate the subsequent discussion of types of literacy.

Background for Literate Thought

Paul and collaborator Wang (Paul, 1998, 2001, 2006; Paul & Wang, 2006a, 2006b) have described literate thought as the ability to think creatively, critically, logically, rationally, and reflectively, especially about information that has been captured, preserved, or stored. This description reflects a predominant focus on the development of cognition by the individual, although it is acknowledged that the social environment (e.g., classroom, school, neighborhood, etc.) plays an important role in contributing to the development of cognition. Literate thought is certainly not a new notion or idea; rather, it is related to or a manifestation of other concepts such as critical thinking or metacognition (e.g., see Calfee, 1994; Olson, 1994; Smith, 1995).

Historically, the concept of literate thought has been influenced by research on orality and the oral tradition (Denny, 1991; Feldman, 1991; Olson, 1989, 1991). More important, it is the research on orality plus the current views on script literacy that have provided us with an emerging and perhaps better understanding of what it means to be literate (for views on literacy, see Beach, 1994; Tierney, 1994; Weaver, 1994).

It is often claimed that script literacy, particularly writing, is responsible for the complexity and abstractness of the mode of thought that is often characteristic of individuals in societies that have high levels of technology and literacy. This condition is purported to result mainly from the capture of the spoken word in print (Denny, 1991; Feldman, 1991; Olson, 1991). On the contrary, there is a growing assertion that reading or writing is not responsible for the development of thought or cognition; rather, these entities are the outcomes of thought. In other words, reading and writing skills are part of the overall language comprehension process. Individuals with a high level of thought can express themselves through the mode of writing or possibly in other literate modes (e.g., speaking, drawing, acting or role playing, etc.).

Writing, or written language, has led to the separation of text and its array of interpretations by individuals who can access print. Thus, with the invention of writing and subsequently the printing press, there now is a separation of information in the text and the reader's interpretation that permits a discussion of the various meanings of the text. Even more important is the fact that information has been captured and individuals can engage in a deeper, more rational and critical reflection of the concept. This leads to or facilitates the production of highly abstract, complex thought because of lessened demands on memory and the ease of refinement and elaboration on the captured text by a mind that is intensely engaged in reflection.

Written language by itself does not lead to a specific development of consciousness—learned or otherwise (e.g., Denny, 1991; Feldman, 1991; Olson, 1994). Writing is an avenue

—similar to mathematics—that can be used to reflect or represent the cognitive products of literate thought. Of course, writing and reading can be used as tools for further developing one's abstract, complex thinking skills; however, they are not the only tools for these purposes.

Based on anthropological data, it can be argued that—similar to script literacy genres, there are oral genres that also represent a separation of text and interpretation, thus inviting reflection and abstraction (e.g., Feldman, 1991; Olson, 1994). For example, in societies with no competing written forms, there are distinctive oral forms that proceed beyond those associated with ordinary colloquial conversations. In this chapter, we are concerned mostly with information that has been captured; however, some attention is given to the value of oral discourse, as discussed later in the section on process drama. The activities used in process drama can also be captured for later discussion and reflection by the students and teacher.

In essence, literate thought develops when individuals have opportunities to reflect on and study captured information—the particular mode of the captured information is not critical. To proceed to high levels of literate thought, individuals need to become familiar with the **metalanguage** (e.g., specialized vocabulary) of the topics or subjects. Finally, as with any other learned activity, it is necessary to acquire and use a bona fide first language at the earliest age possible. In other words, given what we know about thought–language relations, there seems to be a reciprocal relationship between a high level of development in thought and a high level of development in the use of a language (Paul & Jackson, 1993; Quigley & Kretschmer, 1982; Rodda & Grove, 1987).

Types of Literacy

Similar to other controversial educational topics, the term *literacy* has come to mean more than just the ability to read and write or even to refer to print materials. In part, this results from the influence of theories that are predominantly sociocultural in nature (i.e., involving the influences of social and cultural forces) and which have spawned an explosion of literacy terms related to the new literacies or to multiple literacies (e.g., see Bloome & Paul, 2006).

There is no consensus on the manner in which to discuss these new concepts of literacy (e.g., see Bloome & Paul, 2006; Calfee, 1994; Tyner, 1998). One useful framework is that proposed by Tyner (1998), who introduced two broad categorical schemes—tool literacies and literacies of representation—that, unfortunately and unavoidably, overlap in some aspects. Tool literacies refer to the use of technological tools and entail constructs such as computer literacy, network literacy, digital literacy, and technology literacy. Literacies of representation—which is close to our reconceptualized description of literacy as captured information—involve the representation and manipulation of information in entities such as information literacy, visual literacy, and media literacy. There are other examples; consider the following terms: scientific literacy, mathematics literacy, medical literacy, legal literacy, and so on.

If it is accepted that literacy is a form of captured literate information, then three types of relevance here include script literacy (reading and writing), performance literacy (sign or oral literacy), and **caption literacy**. Script literacy simply refers to the traditional practice of reading and writing or to literate information captured in print, reflective of the writing system of society (alphabetic, characters, etc.). Caption and performance literacy are dis-

cussed below. (*Note:* Other types of representations such as Braille literacy, computer and communication boards, alternative communication literacy, and so on are not discussed in this chapter.)

Caption Literacy

In the field of deaf education, teachers and students are familiar with the use of captions—more popularly known as *caption media*—in which print or subtitles accompany films and television programs, typically at the bottom of the screen (or video portion) (e.g., see discussions in Marschark, Lang, & Albertini, 2002; Stewart & Clarke, 2003). Thus, the language of caption media is most likely to reflect the use of colloquial, conversational language used in through-the-air social intercourses. For example, if you watch the television movie *Middlemarch*, you will notice that the structure of conversations and the language used in the movie are not as complex or dense as those that appear in the book by George Elliot (Mary Ann Evans). For the most part, the language used in social face-to-face discourses, such as shorter syntax or sentences and widely known spoken vocabulary, is not as complex as what was used in print. The language used can be more or less complex, depending on the nature of the show; nevertheless, the primary function of media is still entertainment, and this is factored in the selection or development of the monologues and dialogues.

Caption media, as described above, is only one version of our concept of caption literacy. The caption literacy mode can also include the more educational productions (produced for schools) as well as serious videos, which are either audio books or CDs or sign books or DVDs of anything from *The Fox and the Crow* to *Moby Dick* to *A Theory of Everything*.

Developing caption literacy materials for instructional purposes does not seem to be a widespread practice mainly because these types of materials may not be as *entertaining* as caption media. Research on children's comprehension of caption media or caption literacy is limited or virtually nonexistent. Specifically, there is limited research on the comprehension of popular programs using caption media with children who are deaf or hard of hearing (see Ward, Wang, Paul, & Loeterman, 2007). Even more interesting is the growing argument that it is an oversimplification to assume that watching caption media can improve—in wholesale fashion—the ability to read script literacy materials (e.g., see discussions in Loeterman, Paul, & Donahue, 2002; Stewart & Clarke, 2003; Ward et al., 2007). To understand this point, we need to compare caption and script literacy.

Comparison of Caption and Script Literacy

Despite the apparent similarity of the use of *print* in both caption and script literacy, given our current technological limits, it is the manner in which print is used that present major differences between these two modes. For example, the reader of print materials (script literacy) can proceed at a pace that matches his or her style, can reread previous lines, and can even jump ahead to other locations of the text. This provides the important element of reader *control.*

On the other hand, the viewer of caption literacy or media has no control over the rate of the captions that run across the screen. As most caption viewers are painfully aware—sometimes the print dialogue on the screen does not match the utterances of the characters in the particular video frame. This can disrupt the comprehension process, especially if the viewer is looking up at the video and down at the caption periodically.

Look back (i.e., reading the captions again) for the viewer, especially without taping the show, is limited to the amount of captions that remain on screen as well as the length of time that the captions are present on one frame of the screen. Even with repeated viewings, the viewer may not see more than one line or frame at a time because previous captions disappear from the screen. Ironically, one major reason for repeated viewings is to free the individuals from focusing predominantly on the captions so that she or he can enjoy the show.

Caption media and literacy has three major components: video, audio, and print. Thus, access entails the development of skills for all three components, including the ability to handle the juxtaposition or simultaneous occurrence of print, sound, and pictures (e.g., see Stewart & Clarke, 2003; Paul & Wang, 2006a; Ward et al., 2007). The juxtaposition is important because each aspect (print, sound, video) contributes to the message of the show.

Thus, the access skills for caption media or literacy are quite different from those for the traditional script literacy mode as discussed in this text. There might be some overlapping or transferable skills because both modes share the use of print; however, there are differences. For example, with respect to captions, the viewer needs to be aware of the use of caption conventions, which involve the use of character identification (names on the side of the captioned utterance), and the use of parentheses (e.g., for people not on screen or for noises or sounds such as a drum bang, door knock, etc.). Caption conventions are different from print conventions (e.g., use of headings, parentheses, etc.).

Interpretation skills (e.g., making inferences, drawing conclusions, etc.) may be roughly similar for both script literacy and caption literacy or media. The nature of the interpretation is affected by the amount and quality of information in the caption literacy mode as well as by the interaction of several individual variables (e.g., access skills, prior knowledge, and metacognition; the effects of the voices or signs of the speakers or signers; and so on). Although access skills are important, developing literate thought in the caption media or literacy mode still depends on the development of interpretation skills that—in many cases—might need to be a part of classroom instruction. There is a need for further research on the relationship between good caption media or literacy users and good script literacy users as well as on the relations of the *print* conventions of caption literacy to those of script literacy (e.g., Ward et al., 2007).

Performance Literacy

Another type of literacy that may have enormous potential for developing literate thought in children who are deaf or hard of hearing (and other children with disabilities) is performance literacy (e.g., Paul & Wang, 2006a, 2006b). The term **performance** refers to information presented in oral or conversational through-the-air discourses. Examples range from dinner and phone conversations to classroom lectures to process drama to the reading and signing of information that exist in books and other print materials. Performance *literacy* is the capture of this information or exchange; thus, this type of literacy does not contain the use of print as in caption or script literacy.

The concept of performance (not performance literacy) has been influenced by the merits of orality or oral discourse. Information on orality has come from historical research on the oral tradition in both current and preliterate societies (Olson, 1989, 1991, 1994). The use of oral discourse was common for obtaining and discussing information, prior to and, in many cases, after the invention of the printing press. Olson (1989) relates that there were *readers*—individuals whose primary function was to read scripts out loud—who travel to various communities. A crowd would gather and listen to the reader. Only members of the communities participated and, occasionally, someone—often the reader—would be assigned to write or record reactions or responses.

In preliterate societies, individuals had to use their memories to pass on important information to others. In some cases, information was coded in rhyme. That is, one of the ways to remember information was to rhyme the last words of sentences, similar to the lines of a poem. The learning of trades or occupations was conducted primarily through oral discussions and apprenticeships. Thus, to learn to be a blacksmith, an individual would shadow the master and observe as well as listen to the master's explanations of his work. The apprenticeship approach is familiar to many current educators and scholars in professional fields such as medicine, law, music, art, speech and hearing science, social work, and education.

Implications of Performance Literacy

It is easy to demonstrate that the content of information in the performance literacy mode can be as complex and as difficult as information presented in the written mode. The primary example is talking or audio books for the general population or the academic texts prepared for individuals who are blind or visually impaired. Performance literacy materials may contain decontextualized or literate language that closely resembles the vocabulary and grammar of script literacy materials. In essence, it is possible to transliterate all script literacy information electronically, including newspapers or other printed materials such as legal documents and textbooks, into a performance literacy mode (i.e., no print).

It might be easy to convince educators and scholars about the complexity of the information in the performance literacy mode; however, they might remain unconvinced about the practicality of developing literate thought in this mode only in a society such as the United States. We are not advocating that the performance literacy mode should supplant the script literacy one. However, if individuals, particularly children and adolescents who are deaf or hard of hearing, have difficulty accessing script literacy materials, then it might be feasible to transliterate such information in a more accessible mode. Efforts to improve script literacy skills can and should continue and may even be conducted in a parallel fashion along with performance literacy skills.

Individuals need to access such information because of the complexity of concepts and literate language that are present in academic materials. Presenting and capturing information in sign or speech does not make it easier, but it might make it more accessible in the long run because it reduces one level of abstraction (i.e., decoding and understanding the representation of information in print). More important, if information can be presented at or near grade level or at the student's ability level, then the teacher can continue to assist with the development of high-level comprehension and metacognition skills.

Access and Interpretation: Performance Literacy

The access and interpretation skills for script literacy, especially reading, have been the major focus of this book. There are also access and interpretation issues for performance literacy, similar to what was previously discussed for caption literacy. If a teacher uses audio materials only, such as audio books or audio CDs, then students have to develop adequate listening skills to access this form of captured information. Relistening or multiple listenings, similar to multiple readings of scripts, should be encouraged. The teacher will need to employ a mechanism (audiotaping, stopping the tape and taking notes) to assist students in developing study skills, synthesis skills, and so on.

If the teacher uses video materials with *signing* and *sound*, then students need to develop not only viewing skills (i.e., watching the video) but also listening skills (i.e., understanding the dialogues, monologues, etc.). There is an additional aspect: Students should develop the skills to view and listen in a simultaneous fashion. It is no small feat for students to coordinate and synchronize the input from the simultaneous presentation of sound, signs, and captions.

Despite the variations above with respect to access skills, we argue that the interpretation skills (e.g., understanding of the literate language, prior knowledge, metacognitive skills) required for the story or passage in this mode are roughly similar to those interpretation skills relevant to either the print (script) or caption (not as a movie!) mode (e.g., see discussion in Paul & Wang, 2006a, 2006b). Similar to caption literacy, the effects of the speaker or signer, narrator, or characters (e.g., author's or user's voice, style) on individuals' interpretation of the story should be taken into consideration. In fact, this is a much needed area of research. Nevertheless, let us assume that the content is roughly equivalent, for example, for the script literacy passage and its transliterated performance literacy version. In essence, it is possible to develop questions or assign a retell task in classroom situations using the performance literacy mode. The demands for these school exercises are roughly equivalent to what is typically required in classrooms for readers working in a script literacy mode or even in the caption literacy mode.

Instructional Examples

We have attempted to make the case that performance literacy materials can be utilized to perform the same or similar functions as books and other script literacy materials in teaching and learning situations in schools. Children and adolescents who are deaf or hard of hearing can review or study performance literacy materials (i.e., CDs or DVDs) and become engaged in meaningful classroom discussions. Many of our current instructional activities for script literacy can be applied or adapted for performance literacy—specifically, prior knowledge, metacognitive, and assessment activities (e.g., see Paul & Wang, 2006a, 2006b).

Classroom discussions and dialogues can also be videotaped and used to complement existing performance literacy texts that are transliterations of script literacy texts or to complement the use of script literacy materials themselves. For example, in a typical classroom situation, the teacher explains difficult aspects of a topic from a text or dialogues with students via questions and assigned activities. Students also dialogue with each other. Such informational exchanges should be *captured* on videotape or DVD so that the students can relisten or rewatch and reflect on the content of the discussions. This DVD can also become the text for classroom discussion and be used along with script literacy materials in a parallel fashion.

An example of a performance literacy lesson is described in Box 8-1 (Paul & Wang, 2006b, pp. 308–309). As can be seen in Box 8-1, the activities for comprehension instruction are similar to what has been discussed in the use of script literacy materials for reading in this book. It is also important for the teacher to assist children in understanding the structure of the text, to allot time for prestory discussions and for asking prediction and inferential questions about the main aspects of the performance literacy story, and, finally, to encourage children to provide several interpretations of a story.

Another instructional example of performance or performance literacy is discussed in the next section on process drama. Process drama can be used in the performance mode (i.e., live, face-to-face) or in the performance literacy mode (captured on DVD). The advantages of process drama are several; for example, it can contribute to the development and refinement of language use as well as to the development and refinement of cognitive and social skills (McMaster, 1998; O'Neill, 1995; Schneider & Jackson, 2000).

Process Drama

According to Schneider and Jackson (2000), "Process drama is a method of teaching and learning that involves students in imaginary, unscripted, and spontaneous scenes" (p. 38). Unlike a play, process drama is not based on a written script or a fixed scenario but emerges from a theme, event, or text that interests and engages the participants. It involves the creation of a fictional world in which experiences, insights, interpretations, and understandings can be generated and explored. Process drama is not intended for an external audience; rather, participants are an audience to their own efforts (McMaster, 1998; O'Neill, 1995; Schneider & Jackson, 2000).

By nature, process drama is spontaneous, but there is also a need for direction and a plan. Although students have ownership of the process, the teacher must be equipped to guide the students in discovering the predetermined objectives of the lesson. In the classroom setting, the teacher acts as the facilitator, controlling the "episodes" created by the students (McMaster, 1998; O'Neill, 1995; Schneider & Jackson, 2000). The

| BOX 8-1 | **Example of a Performance Literacy Lesson** |

For homework, students are required to watch a signed story about bats on a DVD. The signed story is a transliteration of the printed version included in a reading text. That is, the exact same information has been rendered via the use of signing.

Prior to taking the DVD home, the teacher and students engaged in prestory activities (similar to prereading activities) with the purpose of enriching and activating the students' prior knowledge and background experiences. This type of classroom activity, which has been captured for later use by the students, should motivate students to share their experiences and understanding. Questions that form the basis of the classroom interactions include the following.

Bats: Prestory Questions

The following questions are based on Paul (1998):

1. This is a story about animals called bats. Have you ever seen a live bat? A picture of a bat? Tell me about it. What do you think this story will tell us?

2. Tell me what you know about bats. What do they look like? Are they big or small or both? Are bats different from birds? Why or why not? Are bats similar to birds? Why or why not?

3. What do bats do during the day? At night?

4. Do bats fly in the dark? How do bats fly in the dark? Do bats fly during the daytime? How do they do that?

5. How do people feel about bats? Why? How do you feel about bats? Are bats dangerous? How do you know that?

After watching the DVD at home (or in the classroom), students check their understanding of the story. The DVD includes an exercise that requires retelling and signed comprehension questions such as the following (based on Paul, 1998):

1. What do bats have on their bodies?

2. Why are bats called *mammals*?

3. Are bats dangerous? Why or why not?

4. How do you feel about bats? Do you know more about bats than was presented in this story?

At the next class session, students share their understanding of the story and relate this story to previous stories or experiences. This post-story classroom interaction is captured so that students can refer to and review the sharing of information about the story. The entire lesson and all activities have been conducted without the use of print—that is, in a performance literacy mode.

premise of using process drama as an instructional tool is that it is an active, entertaining way to involve students in the learning process, thereby motivating them to be involved, interested, and creative learners (McMaster, 1998). McMaster promoted process drama as an effective means of supporting every aspect of literacy development including decoding, fluency, vocabulary, discourse, and syntactic and metacognitive knowledge.

Using Process Drama with Students Who Are Deaf or Hard of Hearing Recently, Trezek and Gittings (2008) explored how process drama could address the literacy needs of students who are deaf or hard of hearing. In their discussion, the authors provide concrete examples to illustrate not only how process drama can be applied to teach the phonemic awareness, phonics, fluency, vocabulary, and comprehension skills recommended by the National Reading Panel (2000), but also how this instructional tool could be used to enhance prior knowledge and metacognitive and affective skills. Essentially, these authors suggest that process drama can be utilized to foster the development of skills in both the process and knowledge domains of reading (see Paul 2001, 2003; and Chapter 1 of this text for further discussion). Drawing on instructional activities presented previously in this text, the inclusion of process drama to enhance these activities is described here.

In Chapter 4 of this book, an activity titled *Fishing for Sounds* was described. In this activity, phonemic awareness and phonic skills were taught and reinforced by having students "fish" for a particular sound or word and then blend the sounds to form words. To enhance this activity with process drama, the teacher could begin by asking the students to dramatize the meaning of the word *caught*. Once the activity begins, students could demonstrate the

meaning of the words caught through drama. Using several words (e.g., *man, cat, eat, feed*), the students could create a dramatic episode. It is clear from this example that the teacher would need to preplan and select words not only so that the students could decode them, but also that these words could be used in conjunction with one another to create a realistic scene.

In Chapter 5 of this book, *Sentence Dash* was offered as an activity to promote sentence-level reading fluency. In this activity, students chose a phrase from beginning, middle, and end categories to create sentences to read. By adding a dramatization of the resulting sentence, process drama serves as a means of ensuring that students comprehend the sentences formed. Similarly, the activity *Word Play* described in Chapter 6 already incorporates dramatization to gain understanding of unknown vocabulary. The *Comic Strip* activity explored in Chapter 7, in which students create illustrations of a story in the proper sequence, could be preceded by a dramatic rendition of the story elements.

Process drama activities can also be utilized to build or enhance prior knowledge, develop metacognitive strategies, and support affective skills. If an event cannot be directly experienced, such as through a field trip, then process drama offers an excellent alternative to building prior knowledge of content areas (McMaster, 1998). Engaging in process drama activities also promotes the development of metacognitive strategies. Throughout the dramatization, students are required to answer and generate questions, make predictions, and use mental imagery. Finally, process drama may be an effective means of engaging struggling learners. The motivational, multimodal activities promoted through process drama may be exactly what these learners need to build their self-confidence in an area in which they have traditionally experienced great difficulty. This in turn may provide direct, intrinsic motivation for other reading activities (McMaster, 1998; Trezek & Gittings, 2008). As illustrated here, process drama can be easily incorporated into a variety of literacy instructional activities aimed at improving skills for students who are deaf or hard of hearing.

Summary: Performance Literacy

We have devoted considerable attention to the discussion of performance literacy because we believe that it is an underused entity in education and deafness, especially given the current status of technology. Many students who are deaf or hard of hearing may have extreme difficulty in accessing and using information in script literacy or even in caption literacy if the print element is considered. We suggest that additional means of accessing and interpreting information be used, such as performance literacy, to provide these students with opportunities to learn and to continue to develop their cognitive and metacognitive skills at age-appropriate levels.

Performance literacy should not and cannot supplant script literacy. It provides another avenue for students who are deaf or hard of hearing to work with decontextualized, literate information that is roughly similar to the information in school-based print materials. There is little research to show that performance literacy can facilitate access to the language structures of script literacy. However, students who are deaf or hard of hearing can be exposed to language structures and information at various difficulty levels.

In sum, there has been little empirical research on the merits of using performance literacy materials. Paul and Wang (2006a, p. 35) have suggested that future researchers explore the following list of possible questions:

- What are the contributions of performance literacy to the development of literate thought and as a possible instrument for cognitive development in general?

- What are some possible ways of enhancing and developing performance literacy skills in children and adolescents? Will this improve access to script literacy, particularly the language of print? Will this improve students' understanding of script literacy information?

- What are the implications and effects of using the performance literacy mode in bilingual–bicultural situations?

NEW LITERACIES AND MULTIPLE LITERACIES

It is not an easy task to describe what is meant by *new literacies* and *multiple literacies*, but there is little doubt that this represents a reaction to or shift away from the traditional notion of literacy as reflected by the skills of reading and writing (e.g., see discussions in Bloome & Paul, 2006; Paul, 2006). These new views are the outcomes of emerging social models of literacy, which place more emphasis on how literacy—particularly multiple literacies—is a part of the social and cultural lives of individuals and communities.

These recent views of literacy have spawned research thrusts such as the reading–writing connections, reader-response perspectives, emergent literacy positions, and critical literacy. Although several scholars consider social (or sociocultural) positions to be a paradigm shift from cognitivism (i.e., Chall, Adams, and others as discussed in this text), there are those who view social views as an extension of cognitivism (e.g., see Gaffney & Anderson, 2000; Pearson, 2004). Regardless of the interpretation, it is clear that the focus is different with the employment of terms such as *multiple worlds, multiple ways of knowing* (i.e., epistemologies), and *habits of minds*. More important, the focus is on the development of critical literacy habits, which is taken to mean that readers need to interpret or place the message in the text within a broad context by uncovering hidden agendas, power structures, and social justice issues.

It would not be a stretch to remark that the proponents of new and multiple literacies believe that the current practices of literacy in school (reading and writing) are narrow and oppressive (e.g., see discussions in Bloome & Paul, 2006; Paul, 2006). Academic literacy (i.e., texts) is important—not paramount—and other types of literacies or a variety of literacy sources, especially those that are a part of social worlds of students, should be considered and used as part of the school curriculum. With the implementation of broad literacy practices and multiple literacy genres, students should become more engaged in the meaning-making process. Furthermore, students should recognize that other interpretations (i.e., different voices) are *equally* as important as the so-called expert or predominant culture positions. This reaction also extends to the use of tests that seem to reflect only the views—often called *hegemonic* views—of the mainstream culture.

At first blush, it seems that these new ideas have little to do with the specific development of reading and writing skills as advocated by the National Reading Panel (2000) and much of the information offered in this text. Indeed, there have been harsh criticisms of these narrow, inaccurate practices (i.e., teaching of skills) with respect to the understanding of what it means to be literate (e.g., see discussions in Olson, 1994; Paul, 2006; Pearson, 2004). The assumption has been that the current method of teaching literacy in schools does not prepare students for a diverse, changing world in which they are expected to

work collaboratively and become critical thinkers of information from a variety of sources.

Some of the values promoted by the new and multiples literacies such as collaboration, critical thinking, and multiple perspectives are also shared by traditionalists (for lack of a better word to describe this latter group). There is no doubt that school literacy practices need to be improved, especially the way comprehension has been viewed and assessed (e.g., see the discussions in Paris & Stahl, 2005). In this text, we have maintained that there is a need to provide opportunities for students who are deaf or hard of hearing to be exposed to several passages or texts, not just to a single passage in one text. In other words, teachers should construct questions that require the students to access several sources to render a critical, reflective answer.

In essence, the authors of this text—as well as other cognitivists—have no concerns with showing how social and cultural forces contribute to the language and cognitive developments of individuals. Nevertheless, we argue that our focus on the findings of the National Reading Panel (2000), despite its limitations, means that there should be attention to the role of cognition in the development of reading (and other knowledge domains). Thus, our view strongly advocates the need for the reader to have access and interpretation *skills* in order to comprehend the message—whether it is from one source or from multiple sources.

With respect to children and adolescents who are deaf or hard of hearing, there have been only a few investigations that have examined social effects on reading comprehension. One strong line of research has been influenced by reader-response theory, particularly children's response to literature (Lemley, 1993; Williams, 1994, 2004; Williams & McLean, 1996, 1997). Within this research paradigm, children engage with a text (typically, reading silently or aloud or listening to others' reading) and share their responses with the teacher or with other children in the classroom. The crux of these activities is to encourage children to recognize similarities and differences among a range of responses to issues or events in the passages. In essence, this should lead to an improvement of reading ability, according to social constructivist mechanisms (i.e., the influence of social interactions and discourses on the meaning-making processes of individuals).

There is a need for further investigations within reader-response or other social views of reading, but we recommend that researchers proceed with caution. In our view, reading is essentially a solitary activity, and individuals at some point need to be able to read alone and independently—especially in reading expository texts such as science, history, and philosophy. If the phrase *reading to learn* has any significance, then it is that an individual has the capacity to access sources of information in an independent manner. There are more interactions and reflections between the independent reader and text or texts than there is or can ever be in any social-learning situation.

We do not mean to downplay the role of the social aspects of reading, particularly during the beginning reading stages. We do think that the social process assists readers not only with understanding and interpretation, but also with determining and clarifying the value of information from multiple sources. Critical readers cannot and should not rely on a single source of information. Nevertheless, solitary reading (and thinking) is far more efficient and extensive at the advanced reading stages for the *reading-to-learn* phenomenon.

There is much more to the new literacies and multiple literacies than has been presented in this section. We have only scratched the surface with respect to the issues of power,

oppression, and social justice. If the goal is to develop critical, literate readers, then, in our view, the challenge for educators is to ensure that children and adolescents who are deaf or hard or hearing have access and interpretation skills so that they can read to learn.

CONCLUSION

The main intent of this chapter was to introduce the reader to the concepts and findings of literate thought and to discuss new and multiple literacies. From one perspective, these topics seem to be outside the purview of the discussion of reading and findings from the National Reading Panel that has motivated much of the content of this text. However, with the reconceptualization of literacy as a form of captured information, it is hoped that the notion of reading or literacy has been placed in a context for our readers. Specifically, we attempted to demonstrate that students who are deaf or hard of hearing need to develop the ability to access and comprehend captured forms of information and to interpret or think critically about such information.

The real goal of reading or of working with any form of captured information is the development of literate thought. The path to this goal should not be confined to one form of literacy—specifically script literacy, or traditional reading and writing skills. This emphasis on traditional reading and writing does not consider the newer models of what it means to be literate, at least from the standpoint of research on both orality and oral cultures.

The emerging concepts of new literacies and multiple literacies have presented challenges for traditionalists with respect to the current practices of school literacy. There is no doubt that schools and universities need to address and resolve these shortcomings. Nevertheless, we maintain that the ultimate goal of literacy education is to assist children and adolescents who are deaf or hard of hearing in the acquisition of skills that will permit them to read to learn.

CHAPTER SUMMARY

- Literate thought is the ability to think in a creative, critical, complex, logical, rational, and reflective manner that involves the use of literate language. It is possible to develop literate thought in any mode of captured information, including nonprint (audio books, video books) and print (script).

- The reciprocal relationship between access and interpretation is similar to the reciprocal relationship between word identification and comprehension for English reading. Access facilitates interpretation, and interpretation facilitates access. The ability to access information does not automatically translate into the ability to comprehend or interpret the content. Interpretation skills (e.g., making inferences and applying concepts) may need to be taught.

- Reconceptualizing literacy as a form of captured information, literacies include script literacy, performance literacy, and caption literacy. *Script literacy* refers to the traditional practice of reading and writing or to literate information captured in print that is reflective of the writing system of

society. *Caption literacy* refers to the use of print (or subtitles) that accompanies films and television programs. The language of caption media is most likely to reflect the use of colloquial, conversational language used in through-the-air social intercourses. The term *performance* refers to information presented in oral or conversational through-the-air discourses. *Performance literacy* refers to the captured of this information; there is no print.

- Performance literacy materials can be used to perform the same or similar functions as books and other script literacy materials in teaching and learning situations in schools. Process drama can be used in the performance mode (i.e., live, face to face) or in the performance literacy mode (captured on DVD). Performance literacy should not and cannot supplant script literacy. It provides another avenue for students who are deaf or hard of hearing to work with decontextualized, literate information that is roughly similar to the information in school-based print materials.

- New and multiple literacies represent a reaction to or shift away from the traditional notion of literacy as enacted by the skills of reading and writing. Proponents of new and multiple literacies believe that the current practices of literacy in school (reading and writing) are narrow and oppressive.

REVIEW QUESTIONS

1. What is the authors' definition of *literate thought*? Is literate thought only possible via the skills of reading and writing? Why or why not?

2. In this chapter, the authors presented a categorical framework developed by Tyner with respect to types of literacies. Discuss this framework. How does this framework

relate to the authors' reconceptualization of literacy? How does it relate to the three types of literacies—script, caption, and performance—that are discussed in this chapter?

3. Describe the three types of literacies—script, caption, and performance. How are they similar? How are they different? Consider this question with respect to the concepts of access and interpretation.

4. What is process drama? How is it related to the concepts of performance or performance literacy?

5. What are some of the basic tenets or arguments of the new and multiple literacies with respect to current school literacy practices?

REFLECTIVE QUESTIONS

1. Is it possible to develop literate thought via a nonprint mode in a society such as that in the United States? Why or why not?

2. Now that you have read this much of the text, has your description or definition of literacy changed? Do you think that literacy should be viewed as either a social or cognitive process? Why or why not? What is your understanding of the concerns of the authors of this text with the new and multiple literacies?

APPLICATION EXERCISES

1. Select a chapter from this book and record the chapter on a CD or audio tape (either you or one of your classmates can read out loud). Ask a classmate to develop 5 new questions about the chapter (but do not let him or her show you the questions!). Ask your classmate to read the questions on an audiotape and type them on a sheet of paper. Now perform the following exercise: Listen to the chapter first and then answer the audiotaped questions. If necessary, you can relisten multiple times if necessary. Now read the chapter (again!) and answer the questions in print. Describe your experiences and share them with your classmate and instructor. Help your classmate perform the same activity with different questions (and, perhaps, with a different chapter).

2. Choose a topic or concept and designate a specific grade level of students who are deaf or hard of hearing. Keeping these two elements in mind, create a lesson that utilizes process drama to build background knowledge of the topic, teach specific vocabulary, and assess comprehension. In your lesson plan, briefly describe your topic and then provide an outline that details the concepts, vocabulary, and comprehension strategies you will emphasize during the process drama activity. In addition, include an explanation of how you as the teacher would facilitate the students during the dramatization.

SUGGESTED READINGS AND RESOURCES

Barton, D. (1994). *Literacy: An introduction to the ecology of written language.* Cambridge, MA: Blackwell.

Flannery, K. T. (1995). *The emperor's new clothes: Literature, literacy, and the ideology of style.* Pittsburgh: University of Pittsburgh Press.

Korner, S. (1970). *Categorical frameworks.* Oxford, England: Oxford University Press.

Norris, S. (1992). (Ed.). *The generalizability of critical thinking: Multiple perspectives on an educational ideal.* New York: Teachers College, Columbia University.

Olson. D., & Torrance, N. (1996). (Eds.). *The handbook of education and human development: New models of learning, teaching and schooling.* Cambridge, MA: Blackwell.

REFERENCES

Anderson, R., Hiebert, E., Scott, J., & Wilkinson, I. (1985). *Becoming a nation of readers: The report of the commission on reading.* Washington, DC: The National Institute of Education and The Center for the Study of Reading.

Bartine, D. (1989). *Early English reading theory: Origins of current debates.* Columbia, SC: University of South Carolina Press.

Bartine, D. (1992). *Reading, criticism, and culture: Theory and teaching in the United States and England, 1820–1950.* Columbia, SC: University of South Carolina Press.

Beach, R. (1994). Adopting multiple stances in conducting literacy research. In R. Ruddell, M. Ruddell, & H. Singer (Eds.), *Theoretical models and processes of reading* (4th ed.) (pp. 1203–1219). Newark, DE: International Reading Association.

Bloome, D., & Paul, P. (2006). (Eds.). Literacies of and for a diverse society. Special issue. *Theory into Practice, 45(4).*

Calfee, R. (1994). Critical literacy: Reading and writing for a new millennium. In N. Ellsworth, C. Hedley, & A. Baratta (Eds.), *Literacy: A redefinition.* Hillsdale, NJ: Erlbaum.

Chall, J. S. (1996). *Stages of reading development.* (2nd ed.). New York: McGraw-Hill.

Denny, J. P. (1991). Rational thought in oral culture and literate decontextualization. In D. Olson & N. Torrance (Eds.), *Literacy and orality* (pp. 66–89). New York: Cambridge University Press.

Feldman, C. (1991). Oral metalanguage. In D. Olson & N. Torrance (Eds.), *Literacy and orality* (pp. 47–65). New York: Cambridge University Press.

Gaffney, J., & Anderson, R. (2000). Trends in reading research in the United States: Changing intellectual currents over three decades. In M. Kamil, P. Mosenthal, P.D. Pearson, & R. Barr (Eds.), *Handbook of reading research* (Vol. III) (pp. 53–74). Mahwah, NJ: Erlbaum.

Lemley, P. (1993). *Deaf readers and engagement in the story world: A study of strategies and stances.* Unpublished doctoral dissertation, Ohio State University, Columbus, OH.

Loeterman, M., Paul, P.V., & Donahue, S. (2002, February). Reading and deaf children. *Reading Online, 5*(6). Available at www.readingonline.org/articles/art_index.asp?HREF=loeterman/index.html.

Marschark, M., Lang, H., & Albertini, J. (2002). *Educating deaf students: From research to practice.* New York: Oxford University Press.

McMaster, J. (1998). Doing literature: Using drama to build literacy. *Reading Teacher, 51,* 574–585.

National Reading Panel. (2000). *Report of the National Reading Panel: Teaching children to read—An evidence-based assessment of the scientific research literature on reading and its implications for reading instruction.* Jessup, MD: National Institute for Literacy at EDPubs.

Olson, D. (1989). Literate thought. In C. K. Leong & B. Randhawa (Eds.), *Understanding literacy and cognition* (pp. 3–15). New York, NY: Plenum Press.

Olson, D. (1991). Literacy and objectivity: The rise of modern science. In D. Olson, & N. Torrance, (Eds.), *Literacy and orality* (pp. 149–164). New York, NY: Cambridge University Press.

Olson, D. (1994). *The world on paper.* Cambridge: Cambridge University Press.

O'Neill, C. (1995). *Drama worlds: A framework for process drama.* Portsmouth, NH: Heinemann.

Paris, S., & Stahl, S. (Eds.). (2005). *Children's reading comprehension and assessment.* Mahwah, NJ: Erlbaum.

Paul, P. (1998). *Literacy and deafness: The development of reading, writing, and literate thought.* Needham Heights, MA: Allyn & Bacon.

Paul, P. (2001). *Language and deafness* (3rd ed.). San Diego: Singular Thomson Learning.

Paul, P. (2003). Processes and components of reading. In M. Marschark & P. Spencer (Eds.), *Handbook of deaf studies, language, and education* (pp. 97–109). New York: Oxford University Press.

Paul, P. (2006). New literacies, multiple literacies, unlimited literacies: What now, what next, where to? A response to "Blue Listerine, parochialism & ASL literacy." *Journal of Deaf Studies and Deaf Education, 11*(3), 382–387.

Paul, P., & Jackson, D. (1993). *Toward a psychology of deafness: Theoretical and empirical perspectives* (pp. 215–235). Needham Heights, MA: Allyn & Bacon.

Paul, P., & Wang, Y. (2006a). Literate thought and deafness: A call for a new perspective and line of research on literacy. *Punjab University Journal of Special Education* (Pakistan), *2*(1), 28–37.

Paul, P., & Wang, Y. (2006b). Multiliteracies and literate thought. *Theory into Practice: Literacies of and for a Diverse Society, 45* (4), 304–310.

Pearson, P. D. (2004). The reading wars. *Educational Policy, 18*(1), 216–252.

Pearson, P. D., & Fielding, L. (1991). Comprehension instruction. In R. Barr, M. Kamil, P. Mosenthal, & P. D. Pearson (Eds.), *Handbook of reading research* (2nd ed.) (pp. 815–860).

Pearson, P. D., & Hamm, D. (2005). The assessment of reading comprehension: A review of practices—Past, present, and future. In S. Paris & S. Stahl (Eds.), *Children's reading comprehension and assessment* (pp. 13–69). Mahwah, NJ: Erlbaum.

Pearson, P. D., & Stephens, D. (1994). Learning about literacy: A 30-year journey. In R. Ruddell, M. Ruddell, & H. Singer (Eds.), *Theoretical models and processes of reading* (4th ed.) (pp. 22–42). Newark, DE: International Reading Association.

Quigley, S., & Kretschmer, R. E. (1982). *The education of deaf children: Issues, theory, and practice*. Austin, TX: Pro-Ed.

Rodda, M., & Grove, C. (1987). *Language, cognition, and deafness*. Hillsdale, NJ: Erlbaum.

Schneider, J. J., & Jackson, S. A. W. (2000). Process drama: A special space and place for writing. *The Reading Teacher 54(1)* p. 38–51.

Smith, S. (1995). Creative cognition: Demystifying creativity. In C. Hedley, P. Antonacci, & M. Rabinowitz (Eds.), *Thinking and literacy: The mind at work* (pp. 31–46). Hillsdale, NJ: Erlbaum.

Snow, C., Burns, S., & Griffin, P. (Eds.), (1998). *Preventing reading difficulties in young children*. Washington, DC: National Academy Press.

Stewart, D., & Clarke, B. (2003). *Literacy and your deaf child: What every parent should know*. Washington, DC: Gallaudet University Press.

Taylor, R. (1983). *Metaphysics* (3rd ed.). Englewood Cliffs, NJ: Prentice Hall.

Tierney, R. (1994). Dissension, tensions, the models of literacy. In R. Ruddell, M. Ruddell, & H. Singer (Eds.), *Theoretical models and processes of reading* (4th ed.) (pp. 1162–1182). Newark, DE: International Reading Association.

Trezek, B. J., & Gittings, J. M. (2008). *Process drama: An innovative instructional tool to address literacy needs of students who are deaf or hard of hearing*. Manuscript submitted for publication.

Tyner, K. (1998). *Literacy in a digital world: teaching and learning in the age of information*. Mahwah, NJ: Lawrence Erlbaum Associates.

Ward, P., Wang, Y., Paul, P., & Loeterman, M. (2007). Near-verbatim captioning versus edited captioning for students who are deaf or hard of hearing: A preliminary investigation of effects on comprehension. *American Annals of the Deaf, 152(1),* 20–28.

Weaver, C. (1994). Parallels between new paradigms in science and in reading and literacy theories: An essay review. In R. Ruddell, M. Ruddell, & H. Singer (Eds.), *Theoretical models and processes of reading* (4th ed.) (pp. 1185–1202). Newark, DE: International Reading Association.

Williams, C. (1994). The language and literacy worlds of three profoundly deaf preschool children. *Reading Research Quarterly, 29(2),* 125–155.

Williams, C. (2004). Emergent literacy of deaf children. *Journal of Deaf Studies and Deaf Education, 9(4),* 352–365.

Williams, C., & McLean, M. (1996). *Response to literature as a pedagogical approach: An investigation of young deaf children's response to picturebook reading*. Paper presented at the annual meeting of the American Educational Research Association in New York, April.

Williams, C. & McLean, M. (1997). Young deaf children's response to picture book reading in a preschool setting. *Research in the Teaching of English, 31(3),* 59–88.

CHAPTER 9

COMPUTER TECHNOLOGY, TEACHER EDUCATION, AND IMPLICATIONS FOR PRACTICE IN DEAF EDUCATION

The model of teachers as facilitators reflects the new learning environment that is needed for the 21st century.... The major differences between the traditional and new learning environments have been characterized as follows: teacher-centered vs. student-centered learning, single-sense instruction vs. multisensory instruction, single media vs. multimedia, isolated word vs. collaborative work, information delivery vs. information exchange, passive learning vs. active/exploratory/inquiry-based learning, factual knowledge vs. critical thinking, and artificial context vs. authentic context.... To become a reality, the vision of effective teachers preparing 21st century learners requires an additional ingredient—information and communication technologies. If used effectively, such technologies have the potential of changing classrooms from four walls and a door to dynamic, interactive learning portals that are connected to a worldwide community of learners (Johnson & Mertens, 2006, pp. 222–223).

CHAPTER OBJECTIVES

After completing this chapter, the reader will be able to:

- Explicate the National Reading Panel's conclusions regarding computer technology and reading instruction

- Discuss the findings of using computer technology in reading instruction for students who are deaf or hard of hearing

- Explain the conclusions reached by the National Reading Panel relative to teacher education and reading instruction
- Describe recent research conducted in the area of deaf education and teacher preparation
- Discuss the recommendations for improving teacher education and instructional practice

INTRODUCTION

In Chapters 4 through 7 of this text, the conclusions and recommendations of the National Reading Panel (2000) relative to the five recommended areas of instruction—phonemic awareness, phonics, fluency, vocabulary, and comprehension—were explored. In each of these chapters, we also investigated the research in the field of deafness to determine the alignment of current research with these recommended practices. In addition to the five instructional areas, the National Reading Panel also examined the use of computer technology and teacher education as it relates to reading instruction. Computer technology and teacher education are critical in preparing 21st-century learners:

> The vision of a 21st century learner is that of an individual who is an effective, efficient, self-directed, technologically sophisticated, lifelong learner who collaborates with others for the common purpose of generating and using knowledge to address problems that are of value to the communities in which they live. Technology in the education of D/HH children holds the potential to prepare them to be successful in the future. Tied to the use of technology for this purpose are the preparation of new teachers and the support of existing teachers with an understanding of the complexities that they face in their classrooms. (Johnson & Mertens, 2006, pp. 237–238)

In this final chapter of the text, we briefly review the National Reading Panel's (2000) findings in the areas of computer technology and teacher education. The implications of the panel's findings in these two areas relative to the education of students who are deaf or hard of hearing are also presented and discussed.

COMPUTER TECHNOLOGY AND READING INSTRUCTION

In its comprehensive review of the available research, the National Reading Panel (2000) examined studies that involved using computer technology to deliver reading instruction. The major goals of this review were to determine what results have been obtained, explore the potential use of computers to enhance reading instruction, and investigate questions that remain. Despite the increased availability of computer technology and interest in this area, there has been relatively little systematic research conducted on this topic.

A search of current research yielded only 21 studies that met the National Reading Panel's (2000) criteria for review. These studies explored various topics related to the use of computer technology including instruction in vocabulary, word recognition, comprehension, and spelling. However, the majority of studies examined the addition of speech to computer-presented text, whereas several others investigated the use of comprehensive software packages designed to provide instruction on a wide array of reading skills and topics.

Given the diversity of studies included in the sample, it was difficult for members of the National Reading Panel (2000) to render specific instructional conclusions and formulate recommendations. However, the panel did offer several implications for practice. First, it indicated that computers can be used for some reading instructional tasks. In particular, the addition of speech to computer-presented text can be a promising addition to reading instruction. At the very least, computers offer students the opportunity to interact with text more frequently than with conventional instruction alone. Second, the panel reported that word processing also appeared to be a useful addition to reading instruction. Because writing instruction is often incorporated in reading instructional sessions, the panel felt these studies were relevant; however, it was noted that word processing alone was unlikely to make a difference in children's reading achievement. Rather, word-processing instruction must be used in conjunction with other forms of effective reading instruction (National Reading Panel, 2000).

The third implication of computer technology described by the National Reading Panel (2000) was that multimedia computer software can be used for reading instruction. Although many questions remain, there appear to be many students who benefit from multimedia software, particularly the addition of speech technologies. Despite the lack of experimental instructional studies, the panel indicated that the motivational aspects of using computers should not be overlooked. Finally, the application of hypertext and hypermedia, specifically on the Internet, appears to have great potential.

COMPUTER TECHNOLOGY AND STUDENTS WHO ARE DEAF OR HARD OF HEARING

As indicated above, computer technology alone cannot be considered an effective reading instruction strategy; instead, the effectiveness of computer technology in reading instruction should be examined within the context of how well it facilitates instruction in phonemic awareness, phonics, fluency, vocabulary, and text comprehension (National Reading Panel, 2000). In their meta-analysis, Schirmer and McGough (2005) agreed with the findings of the National Reading Panel that computer technology could be a promising tool in reading instruction for students who are deaf or hard of hearing. However, they found little well-established research on instructional interventions in this area other than a series of studies conducted by Prinz and colleagues (see the review in Schirmer & McGough, 2005) in the 1980s. Since 2005, there have been two studies conducted utilizing computer technology in reading instruction for students who are deaf or hard of hearing.

The 25 participants in the first study (Gentry, Chinn, & Moulton, 2004/2005) were 9- to 18-year-old deaf students who (1) were reading on a third- to fourth-grade level, (2) had average IQ, and (3) used sign language (e.g., combination of signed English and American Sign Language, or ASL) as the primary means of communication. The stimuli were third-grade reading level multimedia stories on CD-ROM. Each participant received four treatments in random order: Treatment 1—print only, Treatment 2—print and pictures, Treatment 3—print and digital video of sign language, and Treatment 4—print, pictures, and digital video of sign language. Student outcomes were measured by story retelling scores. The result showed that students' levels of comprehension in Treatment 2 were the highest, followed by Treatments 4, 3, and 1. The researchers found no statistically significant difference between the presentation of print plus pictures and that of print plus pictures plus sign language. They concluded that the use of pictures significantly assisted the comprehension of written text; however, the effectiveness of adding sign language needed further investigation.

In another study (Wang, Paul, & Loeterman, 2008), a convenient sample was used of 5 teachers and 24 students between 7 and 11 years old who had moderate to severe hearing loss. The intent of this study was to evaluate the effectiveness of a technology-infused project titled the *Cornerstones Approach*, which focused on a deep understanding of a story through word study with specific attention to word-recognition skills and to the development of background knowledge. The *Cornerstones* literacy objectives for students were to (1) recognize a large body of vocabulary words in print, (2) learn about words conceptually and understand multiple aspects of each word, and (3) increase background knowledge to facilitate the comprehension of written materials.

Each *Cornerstones* unit was built around an animated story taken from Public Television's literacy series *Between the Lions*. Digital media technologies made it possible for *Cornerstones* to present different versions of the animated story to accommodate children's different communication methods—ASL, Signing Exact English (SEE II, a system that presents English morphologically), and Cued Speech. *Cornerstones* also provided an online storybook and a hypertext version of the story. Other technology materials supported comprehension and vocabulary objectives and gave teachers a captivating way to spend considerable time on literacy lessons using enhancements such as story maps, graphic organizers, character templates, a large bank of clip art, various computer games, and so on. All *Cornerstones* materials (except the television program), including lesson guides, digitized videos, supporting interactive activities and materials, and lesson plans were freely available on the Web (http: //pbskids.org/lions/cornerstones/) and could be accessed in the classroom or the home (Wang et al., 2008).

The research design of the project involved an alternating treatment design. Two instructional methods—*Cornerstones* and typical (i.e., what was typically used in classroom instruction of reading)—were implemented within subjects. That is, each teacher conducted both *Cornerstones* and typical lessons, and each subject participated in both the *Cornerstones* and the typical interventions. There were three experiments, each of which had two equivalent stories: *Cornerstones* and typical. For assessment, there were two different, but equivalent, sets of pretests and posttests within each experiment, one set per story. For each story, the pretest and posttest were identical. The dependent or outcome variables were word identification, word knowledge, and story comprehension. There were three major components for the qualitative research design triangulation: observations, teacher debriefing, and teacher focus group interviews (Wang et al., 2008).

The results of the study revealed that children who are deaf or hard of hearing demonstrated statistically significant gains from the *Cornerstones* instruction when compared to the typical instruction in all three experiments as measured by word identification and two out of three experiments as measured by story comprehension. The seemingly disappointing results for word knowledge became understandable when the researchers explored the substantial evidence in the implementation data (i.e., the qualitative data), especially the observation checklist conducted by the observers and the teachers. These data supported the existing carryover (i.e., learning) effects in the typical stories in Experiments 2 and 3. Furthermore, the rating artifacts of the word knowledge, assessment fatigue, and the fact that many students disliked being removed from the classroom for testing might also contribute to the indistinguishable difference between the two interventions in word knowledge. Overall, the researchers concluded that the feasibility and perceived value of using the *Cornerstones* approach in the classroom for literacy instruction was overwhelmingly positive (Wang et al., 2008).

In sum, there is a strong need in the field to conduct instructional interventions with larger number of students to further investigate the effectiveness and feasibility of integrating technology and literacy instruction for children who are deaf or hard of hearing. However, it is encouraging to note that the two recently conducted studies reviewed here did explore the use of components of computer technology (e.g., multimedia software packages and hypertext) that the National Reading Panel (2000) also found promising.

TEACHER EDUCATION AND READING INSTRUCTION

According to the National Reading Panel (2000), the evaluation of reading instruction involves four interacting factors: students, tasks, materials, and teachers. Typically, research efforts in this area have focused primarily on students, tasks, and materials. However, recent developments such as class-size reduction and the inclusion of content area standards have necessitated an exploration of the quality of and requirements for teacher education. In fact, **teacher education** and **professional development** were frequently cited areas of concerns during the National Reading Panel's regional hearings.

Teacher education and professional development are two means of acquiring knowledge for teachers. *Teacher education* usually refers to prospective or *preservice* teachers and involves the study of theories and methods of instruction as well as supervised teaching. Once teachers have been inducted into the field, the emphasis shifts from teacher education to professional development for *inservice* teachers. A total of 32 studies met the criteria for the National Reading Panel (2000) review: 11 for preservice teachers and 21 for inservice teachers. Given the differences in time, structure, and continuity of education between these two groups of teachers, members of the National Reading Panel chose to explore these topics separately. A brief overview of the panel's findings in these two areas is provided in the following sections.

Preservice Teachers

The studies conducted with preservice teachers dealt primarily with altering teacher behavior without a conscious focus on student outcomes. The majority of the preservice research reviewed involved early elementary reading instruction. Specifically, these studies explored the following reading topics: (1) comprehension and strategy instruction; (2) general methods of instruction such as Directed Reading-Thinking Activities (DRTA), teaching word-recognition skills,

Directed Reading Activity (DRA), and Informal Reading Inventory; (3) materials; and (4) other topics related to reading such as exploring case studies, study skills, and theoretical orientations to reading (National Reading Panel, 2000).

The vast majority of these studies reported positive results, indicating improved knowledge among preservice teachers. Although the results of these studies were promising, there was no way for the panel to evaluate the transfer of knowledge to effective teaching in the classroom setting because none of the studies reported follow-up data to the treatment condition. In addition, no studies exploring large-scale interventions were included in the National Reading Panel's (2000) sample; therefore, the generalizability of these investigations is limited.

Inservice Teachers

The National Reading Panel (2000) established two primary criteria for their review of studies involving inservice teachers. First, it was essential that student outcome data be reported in these studies. Second, a relationship between changes in teacher behavior and changes in student outcomes needed to be evident in order for the inservice interventions to be considered effective. The 21 studies that met criteria for review were divided into four categories: (1) studies that included both inservice and preservice interventions, (2) studies that measured only teacher outcomes, (3) studies that measured only student outcomes and (4) studies that measured both teacher and student outcomes.

Unlike the preservice studies that were focused primarily on the early elementary levels, the studies of inservice teachers were more equally distributed across grades 1

through 5 and also included a few studies at the secondary level. The focus of the inservice studies were far more eclectic than those conducted with preservice teachers, including such topics as comprehension and strategy instruction, general methods, classroom management, and improving teachers' attitudes. The overall conclusion of studies conducted with inservice teachers indicated that teachers could demonstrate improvements in their teaching and that these improvements had a direct and positive effect on student outcomes. However, as with computer technology, the National Reading Panel (2000) indicated that there was insufficient information to draw specific conclusions about the content of teacher education and professional development. Therefore, both of these areas represent topics for further exploration and research.

TEACHER EDUCATION AND STUDENTS WHO ARE DEAF OR HARD OF HEARING

Although the National Reading Panel (2000) explored the topic of teacher education, this area was not included in the review of the literature titled *Teaching Reading to Children Who Are Deaf: Do the Conclusions of the National Reading Panel Apply?* conducted by Schirmer and McGough (2005). Previous research investigations in this area have employed survey research to collect information on the type of reading materials and instructional methods employed by educators of children and adolescents who are deaf or hard of hearing (Coley & Bockmiller, 1980; Hasenstab & McKenzie, 1981; LaSasso, 1978, 1987). Of particular interest in the context of this book, a study by LaSasso and

Mobley (1997) revealed that a relatively small percentage of these teachers rated their knowledge of reading theory, instructional strategies, and reading materials as up-to-date. Furthermore, the overwhelming majority of teachers of students who are deaf or hard of hearing did not incorporate the teaching of phonology in their reading instruction.

For purposes of this text, we were also interested in learning what research, if any, had been conducted on teacher education for deaf education, particularly those reported since the findings of the National Reading Panel were published in 2000. A search of recent research revealed five survey studies published between 2004 and 2006. One study explored administrators' ratings of the competencies needed to prepare preservice teachers specifically for oral deaf education programs (Lartz & Litchfield, 2005/2006). A second study compared nationally board-certified teachers to nonboard-certified teachers of the deaf or hard of hearing (Scheetz & Martin, 2006). Although these two studies provide insights into the current status of teacher education in the field of deafness, neither study specifically addressed reading instructional practices; therefore, they will not be reviewed. The remaining three survey studies did address topics specifically related to reading instruction for students who are deaf or hard of hearing and, therefore, are reviewed here.

The first study investigated the alignment of early reading instruction (Grades 1–4) to the Wisconsin state standards as well as teachers' perceptions of the standards (Cawthon, 2004/2005). Three participant groups were included in this study: (1) 18 teachers serving only students who are hearing, (2) 8 teachers serving only students who are deaf or hard of hearing, and (3) 10 teachers serving both students who are hearing and deaf or hard of

hearing or in mixed classrooms. This study represented 608 students who are hearing and 135 students who are deaf or hard of hearing, or nearly half (47%) of all students who are deaf or hard of hearing who were educated in the public schools in Wisconsin at the time of this study. Teacher participants in this study were asked to respond to a survey that explored topics in early reading curricula and included many items from the state standards as well as topics specific to working with students who are deaf or hard of hearing. In addition, open-ended questions were included in the survey to gauge the teachers' perceptions of the positive and negative aspects of the standards (Cawthon, 2004/2005).

Although the researcher anticipated variations in responses among the groups of participants, results of the study did not indicate significant differences between the three groups of teachers surveyed. A similar level of alignment between the groups is "an encouraging sign that classroom instruction addresses standards content to the same degree across classroom types" (Cawthon, 2004/2005, p. 431). An evaluation of teachers' responses to the open-ended questions indicated that the teachers serving students who are deaf or hard of hearing only were in most support of the standards because they believed the standards were a way to gain educational equity for their students. These teachers also indicated that guidelines for teaching were an important consideration for standards-based curricula. Teachers serving students who were hearing only were concerned primarily with guidelines for instruction, whereas teachers in the mixed classrooms touched on topics of equity, guidelines for instruction, diversity, and the fact that the standards were politically motivated (Cawthon, 2004/2005).

Teachers in the three groups had varying responses to the negative aspects of the standards. In fact, teachers working with students who are hearing only had vastly different responses than did teachers working with students who are deaf or hard of hearing only. The author was not surprised by this finding given that several categories were included in the survey that related specifically to issues for students who are deaf or hard of hearing (e.g., phonetics and sign language). It is interesting that teachers in the mixed classroom indicated a wide array of responses, echoing concerns from both of the other groups. This led the author to conclude that teachers in the mixed groups equally weighed the needs of both students who are hearing and those who are deaf or hard of hearing (Cawthon, 2004/2005).

In the second study, Teller and Harney (2005/2006) created a 30-item questionnaire to explore the perspectives of program directors on teacher education and instruction for students who are deaf or hard of hearing. Of the 100 surveys randomly distributed to a diverse network of directors (superintendents of residential schools, principals of day school programs, public school programs, etc.), only 19 surveys were returned. Categories in the survey included (1) factors contributing to the quality of a teacher's education, (2) directors' suggestions for changes in programs preparing teachers of the deaf, (3) literacy activities (reading and writing), (4) classroom-management strategies, (5) use of hearing aid and cochlear implant technology, (6) use of manual communication within the programs, and (7) an auditory or oral approach. Of particular interest in this context are the directors' perceptions of the factors contributing to the quality of teachers' education, literacy activities, and suggestions for change.

The overall consensus of respondents indicated that a combination of factors such as course work, practicum experiences, and student teaching contributed to the quality of teachers' education. When asked what resource teachers used in reading instruction, 47% reported using children's literature, 26% indicated using a basal reader supplemented by children's literature, 21% used basal readers alone, and 5% used other materials. An inquiry into the types of writing assignments used with students revealed consistent responses that included journal writing, experience stories, dialogue journals, process writing or writers' workshops, TTY and e-mail communication, and a variety of traditional writings such as expository, narrative, descriptive, persuasive, and essays. In addition, the majority of directors reported that students were engaged in writing daily, and slightly more than half (56%) reported teachers reading to students on a daily basis. It also appeared that the language experience approach was widely used by teachers (80%) on at least a weekly basis (Teller & Harney, 2005/2006).

In regards to assessing reading comprehension, directors reported using the following tools: (1) summarizing, retelling, and sharing with peers; (2) literal and inferential questioning, retelling, sequencing pictures and sentences, drawing pictures, writing, using graphic organizers; (3) interviews, book reports, and sustained silent reading logs; (4) written and oral questions; (5) peer discussion and Socratic seminars; (6) statewide reading achievement tests; and (7) the Bader Reading Inventory and the Language Assessment Inventory (Teller & Harney, 2005/2006).

Finally, responses to open-ended questions revealed seven common suggestions for changes in the preparation of teachers serving students who are deaf or hard of hearing:

1. strategies for serving students with multiple needs;

2. meeting the requirement of the No Child Left behind Act;

3. gaining better signing skills, familiarity with Deaf culture, and managing interpreters;

4. improving ability to address mental health issues among students;

5. increasing the emphasis on working with children with cochlear implants;

6. gaining more experience in itinerant and resource settings and a better understanding of the general education curriculum; and

7. providing experience in auditory and verbal techniques (Teller & Harney, 2005/2006).

It is important to note that the generalizability of these findings is limited because of the low response rate of the surveyed individuals.

The final study explored master teachers' responses to the literacy, science, and mathematics practices used in deaf education (Easterbrooks, Stephenson, & Mertens, 2006). For purposes of this text, only the conclusions related to literacy practices are reviewed. Master teachers of students who are deaf or hard of hearing were identified through a database of 74 teachers from a grant project in deaf education called Join Together. Of the 74 teachers, 37 (50%) completed the survey rating instructional practices. Teachers were asked to rate the benefit they believed the practice offered students as well as the likelihood that they would use the practice. Teachers' responses to the 10 instructional strategies related to literacy instruction are summarized here.

In the category of *providing and monitoring independent reading activities*, 86% of the master teachers indicated that the practice was clearly beneficial to most beneficial, and 83% indicated that they were very likely to highly likely to engage in the practice. When asked to rate the practice *writing as a tool to teach reading*, 89% of those surveyed thought the practice was clearly beneficial to most beneficial, and 78% responded that they were very likely to highly likely to engage in the practice. Results in the category of *using content-area reading materials to promote reading comprehension* indicated that 78% felt the practice was clearly beneficial to most beneficial, and 83% were very likely to highly likely to use this practice. When asked to rate the practice of *having students collaborate on activities that promote literacy development*, only 62% thought that this practice was clearly to most beneficial, and 52% indicated that they were very to highly likely to engage in this practice, whereas 20% of teachers responding to the survey suggested that they were least likely to engage or might engage in this practice (Easterbrooks et al., 2006).

More specifically, related to the findings of the National Reading Panel (2000) discussed in this text, when asked to rate *incorporating specific activities and strategies to promote reading fluency*, 76% of teachers indicated that the practice was beneficial and 64% indicated that they would likely use this practice, although questions were raised regarding how to promote fluent reading among students who are deaf or hard of hearing. When rating *teaching vocabulary meaning through semantically based activities*, 89% of teachers indicated that this practice was clearly to most beneficial, and an equal percentage reported that they were likely to engage in this practice. In regards to the practice of *teaching vocabulary meaning through morphographaphemically based activities*, 65% of teachers indicated that this practice was clearly to most beneficial, and 64% reported that they were likely to engage in this practice. However, teachers questioned their lack of preparation and level of proficiency in instructing students in this area. In the category *teaching metacognition skills such as the use of reading strategies*, 89% of teachers indicated that this practice was clearly beneficial to most beneficial, and an equal percentage indicated that they were very likely to highly likely to engage in the practice. When asked to rate the practice *using technology*, 76% of those surveyed thought that the practice was clearly beneficial to most beneficial, and 70% responded that they were very likely to highly likely to engage in the practice (Easterbrooks et al., 2006).

It is interesting that, particularly in light of the information shared in Chapter 3 and 4 of this text, only 46% of teachers believed that the practice of *teaching phonemic awareness and phonics* was clearly beneficial to most beneficial, and a mere 45% indicated that they were very likely to highly likely to engage in the practice, whereas 36% of teachers stated that they were least likely to engage or might engage in this practice. This category received the most mixed ratings of all the literacy categories surveyed. The greatest concern expressed by the teachers surveyed was that they did not have sufficient training to teach phonemic awareness and phonic skills. Many others did not believe that these skills were appropriate for students who are deaf or hard of hearing (Easterbrooks et al., 2006). The authors of this study advised that, "Teacher preparation programs must carefully inform their teachers in training of the importance of phonemic awareness and phonics instruction for orally communicating students who are deaf or hard of hearing and the alternatives for

teaching these skills through visual means, such as Visual Phonics" (Easterbrooks et al., 2006, p. 405). Collectively, the results of these three survey studies provide an excellent foundation for formulating recommendations for improving teacher-education programs, specifically in the area of reading instructional practices, for both preservice and inservice teachers serving students who are deaf or hard of hearing.

RECOMMENDATIONS FOR IMPROVING TEACHER EDUCATION AND INSTRUCTIONAL PRACTICES

In its review of existing literature, the National Reading Panel (2000) offered suggestions for improving teacher education for both preservice and inservice teachers. Results of the available research conducted with preservice teachers indicated improved knowledge among teachers; however, the transfer of this knowledge to affect student outcomes is an area of research that warrants additional attention. Although studies evaluating professional development practices for inservice teachers indicated that increased knowledge among teachers had a direct and positive effect on student outcomes, there was insufficient information available to draw specific conclusions on best practices in this area.

Clearly, the conclusions drawn by the National Reading Panel (2000) also extend to the preparation of both preservice and inservice teachers in deaf education programs. Additional research is needed to explore topics in teacher education and professional development and, more specifically, what practices lead to positive outcomes for students. In addition to the suggestions presented by the National Reading Panel, we propose that additional topics, discussed below, be the focus of improving teacher-education practices for deaf educators in the area of reading.

According to survey results collected evaluating the reading materials and instructional methods employed by teachers of students who are deaf or hard of hearing (LaSasso & Mobley, 1997), a relatively small percentage of teachers rated their knowledge of reading theory, instructional strategies, and reading materials as up-to-date. Much has been learned about reading instruction since the findings of the National Reading Panel (2000) were published, and current legislation such as the Reading First initiative of the No Child Left Behind Act (2004) reflect the application of the panel's findings on practice. Therefore, our first recommendation is that teacher-education programs preparing preservice educators reevaluate their current reading curriculum and redesign instruction to educate students about the findings of the National Reading Panel, the theoretical support for these practices (e.g., Chall, 1996), and the application of these findings to the education of children and adolescents who are deaf or hard of hearing.

In addition to improving teacher education for preservice teachers, our second recommendation is that efforts need to be made to provide professional development to inservice teachers, especially those prepared prior to the published findings of the National Reading Panel (2000). Strategies such as providing online courses should be explored to meet this demand. Furthermore, additional research is needed to evaluate the effects of improved teacher education and increased knowledge of both preservice and inservice teachers on

outcomes for students who are deaf or hard of hearing. The results of the survey research reviewed in this chapter provide an excellent starting point for identifying critical areas of instruction in which to focus efforts.

As the findings of survey research would suggest (Easterbrooks et al., 2006; LaSasso & Mobley, 1997), an area of need is in educating teachers about the role that phonemic awareness and phonic skills play in reading instruction for students who are deaf or hard of hearing. Given that these skills essentially form the foundation on which higher level reading skills are built (Chall, 1996), they are of critical importance. Teacher educators must recognize the importance of these skills and educate their students accordingly. As teachers of the deaf and hard of hearing become increasingly accountable for meeting state standards and for adhering to legislative acts, the knowledge of these practices and how to adapt them to meet the needs of students who are deaf or hard of hearing becomes increasingly important. These areas of need were also substantiated by the findings of recent surveys of both teachers and program directors (Cawthon, 2004/2005; Teller & Harney, 2005/2006).

In addition to phonemic awareness and phonics instruction, there is a need to address the other three areas of instruction (fluency, vocabulary, and comprehension) recommended by the National Reading Panel (2000). As discussed in Chapters 4 through 7, providing students with phonemic awareness and phonics instruction will improve students' word-recognition skills to the point that fluency, vocabulary, and comprehension skills can be integrated into reading instructional sessions. While instruction in phonemic awareness and phonics is occurring, we encourage teachers to explore the variety of avenues presented in this text (e.g., use of graphic organizers, levels of questions from Bloom's Taxonomy, multiple literacies, process drama, and computer technology) to improve students' language skills and oral or sign comprehension skills. Increasing these language skills will prepare students for the cognitive demands they will encounter later while reading. In essence, we recommend that an equal emphasis be placed on both the process and knowledge components of reading discussed earlier in this text so that balanced instruction in these areas can be achieved.

In sum, we would like to reemphasize why it is critical for preservice and inservice teachers—indeed, anyone who is interested in teaching reading—to continue to study and become familiar with research and effective practices and to understand the children with whom they are working. Teachers not only should know about the *psychology of learning* (i.e., understanding students' particular learning styles, etc.), but also should possess a *deep understanding* of the language and reading areas on which they are planning to focus in the classrooms. This deep understanding should enable teachers to predict or see the specific areas in which students are experiencing problems with respect to the overall goals of language and literacy, particularly reading—the focus of this text. These professionals can use an array of ideas, based on sound linguistic and literacy principles, to assist students in overcoming barriers to their understanding. Teachers with a deep knowledge of language and literacy components, for example, can be extremely creative with their suggestions and strategies for students to increase their comprehension of passages or stories. It should not matter whether you are a teacher in a general education program or in a special education one—both the psychology of learning and the deep understanding of the discipline are critical for becoming an effective teacher.

CONCLUSION

The primary goal of this chapter was to explore the final two areas investigated by the National Reading Panel (2000): computer technology and teacher education. As with many of the previous chapters included in this text, the available research in the areas of computer technology and teacher education in the field of deafness was also reviewed to determine the congruency between these two bodies of literature. In addition to these reviews, recommendations for improving teacher education and instructional practices were offered and a summary of the text, conclusions, and direction for future research provided.

CHAPTER SUMMARY

- According to the National Reading Panel (2000), computer technology such as the inclusion of speech to computer-presented text, word processing, multimedia computer software, and the application of hypertext and hypermedia are areas that show promise and warrant further investigation.

- Although there was insufficient information to draw specific conclusions about the content of teacher education for preservice teachers and professional development for inservice teachers, the National Reading Panel (2000) indicated that the vast majority of reviewed studies indicated positive results related to teacher knowledge and outcomes for students.

- According to the review of the literature conducted by Schirmer and McGough (2005), there is little well established research on instructional interventions in using computer technology in reading instruction for students who are deaf or hard of hearing. Two additional studies published since 2005 were reviewed and indicated promise for using multimedia packages with students who are deaf or hard of hearing.

- With respect to recent research conducted in the area of deaf education and teacher preparation, the majority of previous and recent research has employed survey research as a means of collecting information on this topic. The results of three survey studies were reviewed, exploring topics such as teachers' perceptions of state reading standards, perspectives of program directors on teacher education and instruction for students who are deaf or hard of hearing, and master teachers' responses to literacy, science, and mathematics practices used in deaf education. The findings of these studies indicate the need for further exploration in specific areas related to reading instructional practices for both preservice and inservice teachers of students who are deaf or hard of hearing.

- We offered several recommendations for improving teacher education and instructional practices including the following. (1) Teacher education programs should prepare preservice educators to reevaluate their current reading curriculum and redesign instruction to educate students about the findings of the National Reading Panel, the theoretical support for these practices, and the application of these findings to the education of children and adolescents who are deaf or hard of hearing. (2) Professional development should be provided to inservice teachers through strategies such as online courses. (3) Additional research should be conducted to evaluate the effects of improved teacher education and increased knowledge of both preservice and inservice teachers on reading outcomes for students who are deaf or hard of hearing. (4) Both preservice and inservice teachers need to be educated regarding the role that phonemic awareness and phonic skills plays in reading instruction for students who are deaf or hard of hearing and the appropriate strategies for implementing this instruction with students. (5) Methods to improve fluency, vocabulary, and comprehension instruction as well as enhancing prior knowledge and metacognitive strategies need to be included in education for preservice teachers and professional development efforts for inservice teachers serving students who are deaf or hard of hearing.

REVIEW QUESTIONS

1. Based on the findings of the National Reading Panel (2000), what are the five instructional implications relative to computer technology?

2. What were the general conclusions of the National Reading Panel (2000) in regards to teacher preparation for preservice teachers and professional development for inservice teachers?

3. What are the authors' recommendations for improving teacher preparation for preservice teachers and professional development for inservice teachers of students who are deaf or hard of hearing?

REFLECTIVE QUESTIONS

1. Choose a children's short story or content-specific passage. Using this reading as your foundation, describe in detail a plan for utilizing computer technology to enhance instruction of this reading for students who are deaf or hard of hearing at a specified grade or age level.

2. Easterbrooks et al. (2006) surveyed master teachers to gauge their perspectives on 10 reading instructional practices utilized with students who are deaf or hard of hearing. According to their results, the categories of *having students collaborate on activities that promote literacy development, incorporating specific activities and strategies to promote reading fluency, teaching vocabulary meaning through* *morphographaphemically based activities,* and *teaching phonemic awareness and phonics* were areas in which teachers had concerns and questions regarding practices. Choose one of the areas identified above and, using information provided in this text, create a professional development presentation on this topic. Your presentation should include the following elements relative to your chosen area: (a) findings of the National Reading Panel report in this specific area, (b) research conducted in this area for students who are deaf or hard of hearing, (c) ideas for instructional activities, (d) methods of assessment, and (e) directions for future research.

SUGGESTED READINGS AND RESOURCES

Donovan, M., & Bransford, J. (Eds.). (2005). *How students learn: History, mathematics, and science in the classroom.* Washington, DC: National Research Council.

Fenstermacher, G., & Soltis, J. (2004). *Approaches to teaching.* New York: Teachers College, Columbia University.

Noddings, N. (1995). *Philosophy of education.* Boulder, CO: Westview Press.

Phillips, D., & Soltis, J. (2004). *Perspectives on learning.* New York: Teachers College, Columbia University.

REFERENCES

Cawthon, S. W. (2004/2005). Early elementary curricular alignment and teacher perspectives on standards-based reform. *American Annals of the Deaf, 149* (5), 428–435.

Chall, J. S. (1996). *Stages of reading development.* (2nd ed.). New York: McGraw-Hill.

Coley, J., & Bockmiller, P. (1980). Teaching reading to the deaf: An examination of teacher preparedness and practices. *American Annals of the Deaf, 125,* 909–915.

Easterbrooks, S. R., Stephenson, B., & Mertens, D. (2006). Master teachers' responses to twenty literacy and science/mathematics practices in deaf education. *American Annals of the Deaf, 151* (4), 398–409.

Gentry, M. M., Chinn, K. M., & Moulton, R. D. (2004/2005). Effectiveness of multimedia reading materials when used with children who are deaf. *American Annals of the Deaf, 149*(5), 394–403.

Hasenstab, M. S., & McKenzie, C. D. (1981). A survey of reading programs used with hearing-impaired students. *The Volta Review, 83,* 383–388.

Johnson, H., & Mertens, D. M. (2006). New strategies to address old problems: Web-based technologies, resources, and applications to enhance deaf education. In D. F. Moores & D. S. Martin (Eds.), *Deaf learners: Developments in curriculum and instruction* (pp. 221–242). Washington, DC: Gallaudet University Press.

Lartz, M. N., & Litchfield, S. K. (2005/2006). Administrators' ratings of competencies needed to prepare preservice teachers for oral deaf education programs. *American Annals of the Deaf, 150* (5), 433–442.

LaSasso, C. (1978). A national survey of materials and procedures used to teach reading to hearing-impaired children. *American Annals of the Deaf, 123,* 22–30.

LaSasso, C. (1987). Survey of reading instruction for hearing-impaired students in the United States. *The Volta Review, 89,* 85–98.

LaSasso, C. & Mobley, R. T. (1997). National Survey of reading instruction for deaf or hard-of-hearing students in the U.S. *The Volta Review, 99,* 31–59.

National Reading Panel. (2000). *Report of the National Reading Panel: Teaching children to read—An evidence-based assessment of the scientific research literature on reading and its implications for reading instruction.* Jessup, MD: National Institute for Literacy at EDPubs.

No Child Left Behind Act. (2004). U.S. Department of Education. Retrieved December 11, 2007, from http://www.ed.gov/nclb/landing.html.

Scheetz, N. A., & Martin, D. S. (2006). Teacher quality: A comparison of national board-certified and non-board-certified teachers of deaf students. *American Annals of the Deaf, 151* (4), 71–87.

Schirmer, B., & McGough, S. (2005). Teaching reading to children who are deaf: Do the conclusions of the National Reading Panel apply? *Review of Educational Research, 75* (1), 83–117.

Teller, H., & Harney, J. (2005/2006). View from the field: Program directors' perceptions of teacher education and the education of students who are deaf or hard of hearing. *American Annals of the Deaf, 150* (5), 470–479.

Wang, Y., Paul, P., & Loeterman, M. (2008). *Integrating Technology and Reading Instruction with Children Who are Deaf or Hard of Hearing—The Effectiveness of Cornerstones Project.* Manuscript submitted for publication.

EPILOGUE

SUMMARY OF TEXT

The goal of this epilogue is to review the most salient features of each chapter of the book, thereby providing the reader with concise summaries of the entire text. Chapter 1 provided an introduction to reading and deafness, focusing on a discussion of current reading achievement levels and the need to improve reading comprehension assessments to ensure that valid and reliable information is available. We also introduced the process-and-knowledge view (Paul, 2003) as a framework for understanding the reading difficulties of students who are deaf or hard of hearing and provided the rationale for the text. The primary objective of Chapter 2 was to supply an overview of the theoretical orientation that grounded the text (Chall, 1996) and to discuss how this theory applies to reading and deafness. A brief overview of the general findings of the National Reading Panel (2000) was also provided.

The purpose of Chapter 3 was to present the research on phonology and deafness, beginning with a discussion of working memory and its role in the reading process. The evidence that readers who are deaf or hard of hearing, particularly skilled readers, have access to phonological information and can apply this information to reading tasks was also presented and discussed. A description of four alternative methods of acquiring phonology knowledge for individual who are deaf or hard of hearing—speech reading, articulatory feedback, Cued Speech, and Visual Phonics—was given. Many of these concepts were reinforced, explicated, and applied to practice in Chapter 4.

Beginning in Chapter 4 and continuing through Chapter 7, we reviewed in greater detail the findings of the National Reading Panel (2000) for each of the five instructional areas: phonemic awareness, phonics, fluency, vocabulary, and comprehension. We also provided a synthesis of the research available in the field of reading and deafness to explore the alignment between the recommendations of the panel and the instructional strategies currently being utilized with students who are deaf or hard of hearing. A list of assessments for each area of instruction was provided, as well as sample Individualized Education Program (IEP) goals and short-term objectives, an overview of commercially available curricula addressing specific skill areas, and ideas for instructional activities. In each of these chapters, summary statements and suggestions for future research were also offered.

In Chapter 8, we introduced the reader to the concepts of literate thought. We explored three types of literacies, or captured information, including script, caption, and performance literacy. Examples of activities such as process drama that incorporate different types of literacies into reading instruction for students who are deaf or hard of hearing were also provided. Finally, definitions and descriptions of new literacies and multiple literacies were investigated. In Chapter 9, the findings of the National Reading Panel (2000) in the areas of computer technology and teacher education were reviewed. As with Chapters 4 through 7, research conducted in the field of reading and deafness was also reviewed to determine the congruency of practices with the recommendations of the panel. The findings of survey research conducted in deaf education provided specific areas that became the focus of our recommendations for improving teacher education practices. In the following section, we revisit the three assumptions about reading and deafness that we used to guide our discussions throughout the text and offer directions for future research.

CONCLUSION AND DIRECTIONS FOR FUTURE RESEARCH

The first assumption discussed in Chapter 1 was that the English reading development of students who are deaf or hard of hearing is similar to that of students with typical hearing who are reading in English as a first language. In other words, the research indicates that students who are deaf or hard of hearing proceed through developmental stages, make errors, and use general reading strategies that are roughly similar to those of children who have typical hearing. This view, labeled the *qualitative-similarity hypothesis* (Paul, 2001, 2003), was described in detail in Chapter 1. We also provided an overview of the cognitive–interactive information-processing theory (Chall, 1996) and the findings of the National Reading Panel (2000) that support this theoretical orientation to reading.

Throughout our discussion of the five recommended areas of instruction (National Reading Panel, 2000) included in Chapters 4 through 7, we provided alternative means of delivering this instruction to meet the unique needs of students who are deaf or hard of hearing. We implore professionals who are preparing teachers in the field of reading and deafness as well as classroom teachers to become familiar with the theoretical underpinnings of the practices recommended by the National Reading Panel (2000), as well as the research supporting these practices, and to continue to evaluate the application of these practices to reading instruction for students who are deaf or hard of hearing. Research efforts in this area can evaluate the effectiveness of educating both preservice and inservice teachers on the importance of these topics as well as the effects of increased knowledge among teachers on student outcomes.

Our second assumption was that there is a strong reciprocal relationship between the conversational-based form (i.e., spoken or signed) and the written-based form (i.e., print or written language) of the same language—in this case, English. This requires that children have a working knowledge of the components of English while learning to read English. This has been supported by the strong relationship between phonemic awareness, phonics, and the development of beginning reading skills. In essence, this reciprocal relationship reflects the notion of a 'balanced' approach to the development of reading as advocated by the National Reading Panel (2000) and others (e.g., Pearson, 2004). Students need skills in both word identification (e.g., phonemic awareness and phonics) and comprehension (e.g., vocabulary, prior knowledge, and metacognition) to develop beginning and advanced reading ability. Word identification facilitates the development of comprehension, and comprehension facilitates the development of word identification.

As discussed extensively in Chapters 3 and 4 and touched on again with regard to teacher education practices in Chapter 9, there is a critical need for teachers of students who are deaf or hard of hearing to understand the importance of developing phonemic awareness and phonic skills as well as the strategies for adapting these practices using alternative methods such as Visual Phonics. Research efforts in this area need to continue and be expanded to explore the effects of developing phonemic awareness and phonics skills, particularly as they relate to the acquisition of other reading skills such as fluency, vocabulary, and comprehension. Additional research efforts can focus on the specific training requirements necessary to effectively implement phonemic awareness and phonics skill instruction with students.

The third and final assumption that guided this text is that we believe that it is necessary to teach reading skills explicitly in meaningful, structured situations. Throughout this text, we have offered examples of effective instructional strategies as well as reviews of commercially available curricula and assessments that can be utilized by teachers to provide systematic and explicit reading instruction for students who are deaf or hard of hearing and to evaluate the results of their efforts through assessment. Future research thrusts in this area can concentrate on identifying curricular interventions and the adaptations required to effectively implement curricula with students who are deaf or hard of hearing. We also believe that there is a pressing need to identify or create valid and reliable assessments to gauge the effectiveness of practices and interventions.

GLOSSARY

A

access: The ability to decode words in print that involves, among other factors, the need for fluent and accurate word-identification skills. There is a reciprocal relationship between access and interpretation in reading. See also *interpretation*.

American Sign Language: Also referred as ASL, a visual-gestural language in North America that is particularly structured to accommodate the visual capacities of the eye and motor capabilities of the body. It has two major characteristics: visual-gestural and rule-governed. It entails both manual and nonmanual features. The manual features pertain to the shapes, positions, and movements of the hands, whereas the nonmanual features refer to the movement of the cheeks, lips, tongue, eyes, eyebrows, shoulders, and the body (e.g., for body shifts). Most of the information in ASL is presented and conveyed in front of the signer's body. Signers communicate by executing systematic manual and nonmanual body movements. Space and movement play important linguistic roles in ASL.

articulatory feedback: For individuals who are deaf or hard of hearing, the tactile-kinesthetic feedback system is used to gain phonological information about print. See *tactile-kinesthetic feedback system*.

automaticity: The ability to read individual words accurately and quickly.

B

base words: Words from which many other words are formed.

Bilingual/Bicultural (Bi-Bi): Programs supported by the notion of a Deaf epistemology, where instruction is delivered through ASL, mostly in a classroom similar to what exists in residential schools, and the goal of the program is that the students are truly bilingual and bicultural. Students in these Bi-Bi programs would not only learn the common curriculum of hearing students, but also study the history of Deaf culture and Deaf community.

Bloom's Taxonomy: A model that divides objectives and skills for student learning into three domains: affective, psychomotor, and cognitive. It is hierarchical in nature—that is, the acquisition of skills at the higher levels depends on prerequisite knowledge and mastery of lower-level skills. It was first proposed in 1956 by Benjamin Bloom, an educational psychologist at the University of Chicago. The original goal of Bloom's Taxonomy was to encourage educators to focus skill development in all three domains, thereby creating an increasingly holistic form of education.

C

caption literacy: Refers to the use of print (or subtitles) that accompanies films and television programs. The language of caption media is most likely to reflect the use of colloquial, conversational language used in through-the-air social discourse. It is an oversimplification to assume that watching caption media can improve the ability to read script literacy materials.

cochlear implant: A surgically implanted electronic device that directly stimulates any functioning auditory nerves inside the cochlea to provide a sense of sound for individuals who are profoundly deaf or severely hard of hearing.

cognitive-interactive view: A reading model under the category of cognitive models. Advocates of the cognitive-interactive view believe that a reader is an active information processor and that reading comprehension is driven by the reader's prior knowledge as well as information from the text. It is held that construction of meaning requires the development and coordination of both bottom-up and top-down skills.

comprehension: The ability to obtain meaning from written text for some purpose. Comprehension is the primary goal of reading.

Conceptually Accurate Sign English (CASE): See *signed English.*

contact signing: See *signed English.*

content words: Nouns, verbs, and adjectives, as well as most adverbs, that have a definable meaning.

criterion-referenced tests: Formal assessments that compare a student's test score against a preestablished criterion or benchmark. Criterion-referenced assessments have nothing to do with how others performed on the same test. They are useful for mastery-level learning or competency-based assessment.

Cued Speech: Also referred to as *Cued Speech/Language,* a sound-based, visual communication system that uses eight handshapes in four different locations in combination with the natural mouth movements of speech. During cuing, the speaker keeps his or her hand near the mouth while speaking. Thus, speech reading is completed by adding discriminating information (i.e., the manual gestures or cues). The emphasis is on visually representing the sounds of spoken language—that is, delivering complete phonological information. Cued Speech was initially developed to help deaf children decode speech by eliminating speech reading ambiguities to further assist their language and literacy development in English. It has now been adapted to more than 56 languages. Cued Speech is neither a language nor a philosophy; it is a communication system.

D

deaf: Individuals who have severe (70 to 89 decibels) or profound (90 decibels or greater) hearing loss.

Deaf community: A community within Deaf culture. It neither automatically includes all individuals with hearing loss nor excludes any hearing individuals. A person is Deaf if he or she identifies himself or herself as a member of the Deaf community and is accepted by other members as a part of the community. Hearing individuals, such as people who attend deaf schools, children of deaf adults (CODA), and sign language interpreters, can be included in the Deaf community as well.

Deaf culture: A culture in which deafness is considered as a difference in human experience rather than a disability. The word *deaf* is often capitalized in writing and referred to as "big D Deaf." The primary languages of individuals who identify themselves as Deaf are sign languages.

Deaf epistemology: A worldview or knowledge framework that is uniquely attributed to Deaf individuals which is analogous to the notion of a feminist epistemology.

E

expressive sign vocabulary: The words we use when we sign.

F

figurative language: Speech or writing that departs from literal meaning in order to achieve a special effect or meaning—that is, speech or writing that employs figures of speech (e.g., fixed idioms) such as similes (*She smiles like a flower*), metaphors (*The tree is an umbrella*), and idiomatic expressions (*It was raining cats and dogs*).

finger spelling: Also referred as *dactylology,* a code that represents the letters of the English writing system through hand shapes and positions.

Flesch-Kincaid readability statistic: A feature from the Microsoft Word program that uses the number of words per sentence and number of syllables per word to calculate a grade-level readability for a given passage.

fluency: The ability to read a text accurately and quickly with proper expression.

function words: Include determiners (*the, a, an*), prepositions (*in, on, by*), conjunctions (*and, but*), pronouns (*it, he, they, that which*), and auxiliary verbs and copulas (*can, is, would*), and so on.

G

graphemes: The smallest units of written language—that is, letters.

graphic organizers: Also known as *maps, webs, charts, graphs, frames,* or *clusters,* they use diagrams or other pictorial devices to illustrate concepts and interrelationships among concepts in a text.

H

hard of hearing: Individuals with slight (27 to 40 decibels), mild (41 to 54 decibels), or moderate (55 to 69 decibels) hearing loss.

hearing impairment: A generic term referring to all types, causes, and degree of hearing loss. An individual's hearing threshold level is indicated on the audiogram as a *pure-tone average* (PTA), unaided, across a range of speech frequencies (500, 1000, 2000 Hertz). The pure-tone audiogram is designed to chart hearing sensitivity from 0 dB to 110 dB.

I

independent reading level text: Text that is relatively easy for the reader and can be read with 95% accuracy.

instructional reading level text: Text that is challenging but manageable for the reader and can be read with 90% accuracy.

International Phonetic Alphabet (IPA): A system of phonetic notation based on the Latin alphabet to represent the sounds of spoken language.

interpretation: Entails understanding what one has read and then using that information during selected tasks such as making inferences within and across passages, stating your views on the topic, or critically evaluating the truthfulness of the information. Interpretation is dependent on access skills. There is a reciprocal relationship between access and interpretation in reading. See also *access*.

K

knowledge of alphabetic principle: The awareness that words are composed of letters that are related to phonemic segments (e.g., phonemes) from spoken language or, in other words, the awareness that written spellings systematically represent spoken words.

L

listening vocabulary: The words we need to know to understand what we hear.

literacy: Traditionally and historically, *literacy* has been defined as the ability to read and write via comprehension and interpretation or the construction of meaning. It is now called a *narrow* (or *limited*) *perspective of literacy* (or *reading*), or *script literacy*.

literate information: Refers to the style of information that has been presented in print materials—namely, abstract, complex, and removed from context or otherwise decontextualized information.

literate thought: The ability to think creatively, critically, logically, rationally, and reflectively, especially about information that has been captured, preserved, or stored.

M

manually coded English systems: Sign-based communication systems that attempt to represent the structure of English, particularly English words and word parts, and provide an avenue for parents to learn and use signing without learning a new language. Manually coded English systems include the Rochester method, Seeing Essential English (SEE I), Signing Exact English (See II), signed English, manual English, Conceptually Accurate Sign English (CASE), Pidgin Sign English, and contact signing.

metacognition: Also called *comprehension monitoring*, it refers to thinking about thinking.

metalanguage: A language used to discuss other languages. More broadly, *metalanguage* refers to any terminology or language that is used to make statements about language itself.

metalingustic: Related to thinking about language.

miscue analysis: Coined by Goodman in 1969 to be the alternative preferred term to *mistake* or *error*. The underlying premise of the miscue analysis is that the miscues students produce are neither accidental nor random, but rather indicate the students' language and personal experiences. Once the student has completed the passage reading, each miscue is analyzed to determine if it was related to the context (either proceeding or following), preserved the essential meaning, and whether or not the student corrected the miscue. This method allows the rater to determine both the quantity and quality (i.e., type) of miscues that occurred during passage reading.

morphemes: The smallest meaningful units of a language.

morphology: The internal structure of words.

N

new literacies and multiple literacies: Represents a reaction to or shift away from the traditional notion of *literacy* as reflected by the skills of reading and writing. Reconceptualizing *literacy* as a form of captured information, literacies include script literacy, performance literacy, and caption literacy.

nontransfer studies: Studies that measured participants' ability to fluently read and comprehend a passage after repeated exposures to the same passage were provided.

norm-referenced assessments: Formal assessments that compare one student's performance with what might be normally expected of other students. Norm-referenced assessments are useful in determining the overall developmental level of a student with respect to others.

O

oral vocabulary: Words we know and use in spoken language.

oralism: A practice in education of students who are deaf or hard of hearing in which the major emphasis are speech, speech reading (i.e., lip reading), and auditory training or learning. There are two major groups of approaches: unisensory and multisensory. In unisensory approaches, the major emphasis is on developing audition; it can be described as auditory, aural-oral, aural, auditory-verbal, acoupedic, acoustic, and auditory global. The multisensory approaches involve the use of both audition and vision in a roughly equal manner. It may also include a tactile component and is labeled as the auditory-visual-tactile technique. Cued Speech/Language is an example of multisensory approach.

orthography: Defines the sets of symbols used and the rules on how to write these symbols in written languages.

P

performance: Refers to information presented in oral or conversational through-the-air discourses.

performance literacy: The capture of information through speech or signing.

phonemes: The smallest units of sounds. Phonemes are the building blocks of languages.

phonemic awareness: The ability to notice, think about, and work with the individual sounds in spoken words. Skills in this area usually develop after general phonological awareness and typically requires instruction.

phonics: Letter–sound correspondence or grapheme–phoneme correspondence. Simply put, phonemic awareness skills typically involve the manipulation of phonemes in spoken language without the aid of print.

phonological awareness: A general awareness of the sound system of a language. Children recognize that spoken language contains structures that are separate from meaning. By focusing on the internal structures of words, children can hear or recognize chunks of sounds such as syllables and rhymes.

phonology: Refers to the sound structure of speech in spoken languages. Particularly, it is related to the perception, representation, and production of speech sounds. The phonological aspects of language include its prosodic dimensions (e.g., intonation, stress, and timing) and its articulatory units (e.g., words, syllables, and phonemes).

Pidgin Sign English (PSE): See *signed English.*

pragmatics: The study of language use.

prefixes: Word parts that are "fixed" to the beginnings of words.

prior knowledge: Includes (1) passage-specific prior knowledge that refers to knowledge about the language elements or text information and (2) topic-specific prior knowledge that reflects information that is either not explicitly in the text or cannot be inferred from the existing text information.

process drama: A method of teaching and learning that involves students in imaginary, unscripted, and spontaneous scenes. Unlike a play, process drama is not based on a written script or a fixed scenario but instead emerges from a theme, event, or text that interests and engages the participants. It involves the creation of a fictional world in which experiences, insights, interpretations, and understandings can be generated and explored. Process drama is not intended for an external audience; rather, participants are an audience to their own efforts.

process-and-knowledge view: A perspective that asserts that there is a reciprocal relation between the processing of print and an understanding or interpretation of the information. The emphasis is on this reciprocity—the process domain facilitates the use of the knowledge domain, and the knowledge domain facilitates the better use of the process domain. *Processing print* refers to access skills such as the use of word identification and larger discourse (e.g., phrases and sentences) processes as well as the ability to convert print—typically via the use of a phonological code—for the purpose of constructing meaning in the head. The goal is for processing to become automatic so that much of the reader's energy and resources can be used to comprehend and interpret the text. The *knowledge domain* refers to prior knowledge of the story (including the language of print) and other broadly related topics, metacognitive skills (including inferential skills), and awareness of the social and contextual frameworks of the story. The knowledge domain also includes aspects of critical reading.

professional development: Continuing education for *inservice* teachers.

pseudoword: A unit of speech or text that seems like an actual word in a certain language but, in fact, is not part of the lexicon. Pseudoword still respects the phonotactic restrictions of the language that distinguishes pseudowords from nonwords. For example, "boh" is a pseudoword in English while "bdf" is an example of a nonword.

R

reading vocabulary: Words we know and use in print.

receptive sign vocabulary: The words we need to know to understand the signs we see.

Rochester method: A manually coded English system in which finger spelling and speech are used simultaneously.

root words: Words from other languages that are the origins of many English words.

S

script literacy: The capture of information through print or written symbols—that is, reading and writing. See also *literacy*.

Seeing Essential English (SEE1): A similar manually coded English system as Signing Exact English (SEE2). Compared with SEE2, SEE1 uses more invented sign markers and more signs to represent a word, whereas SEE2 incorporates an ASL sign if it translates into only one English word as much as possible.

semantic organizers: Also referred to as *semantic maps* or *semantic webs*, these graphic organizers look similar to a spider web—that is, lines connect a central concept to various related ideas and events.

sign vocabulary: The words we use or recognize in signing.

signed English (SE): A manually coded English system that is the least representative of English. The term is often used interchangeable with *English signing, contact signing, Conceptually Accurate Sign English (CASE),* and *Pidgin Sign English (PSE)*.

Signing Exact English (SEE2): One of the most widely used manually coded English systems in educational programs for students who are deaf or hard of hearing. It incorporates more ASL signs (i.e., ASL-like signs) than Seeing Essential English (SEE1); meanwhile, it is more representative of English than English Signing or Signed English. For example, in Signing

Exact English, *indescribable* will be signed as IN-DESCRIBE-ABLE.

Simple View of Reading: A perspective that argues for assessing word recognition, phonemic awareness, and text comprehension of narrative and expository passages to measure reading achievement. Much of the focus of the Simple View is on decoding and text comprehension. The Simple View seems to emphasize the accessing and comprehension of a single passage (i.e., passage specific information), whereas a broader view is concerned with factors such as prior knowledge (topic *and* broad knowledge), metacognition, and attitude (engagement), which can impact both decoding and comprehension. The broader view advocates the use of several passages on comprehension tests.

speaking vocabulary: The words we use when we speak.

speech reading: Previously referred to as *lip reading*, refers to the process of understanding a spoken message through observation of the speaker's face.

suffixes: Word parts that are "fixed" to the ending of words.

syntax: Also referred to as *word order* or *sentence organization*, it is the rule of a language that shows how the words should be arranged to form a sentence.

T

tactile-kinesthetic feedback system: Refers to mouth movements combined with vocal sensations (e.g., voiced, unvoiced, etc.) produced to represent each phoneme.

Taxonomy of Educational Objectives: See *Bloom's Taxonomy*.

teacher education: Refers to prospective or *preservice* teachers and involves the study of theories and methods of instruction as well as supervised teaching.

Total Communication (TC): An approach or philosophy that intends to utilize many modes of communication such as signed, oral, and auditory, as well as written and visual aids, depending on the particular needs and abilities of students who are deaf or hard of hearing. In practice, most Total Communication programs use some form of Simultaneous Communication (SimCom).

transfer studies: Studies that measured the ability of participants to generalize or transfer the gains achieved on fluently reading or comprehending one passage to the ability to fluently read or comprehend a new or novel passage.

V

Visual Phonics: The abbreviated title for See The Sound/Visual Phonics (STS/VP), which is a multisensory system consisting of 46 hand cues and corresponding written symbols that represents aspects of the phonemes of a language and the grapheme–phoneme relationships (phonics). Visual Phonics was originally designed as a reading instructional tool for teaching letter–sound correspondences with the assumption that Visual Phonics use would fade when the students began to internalize the relationships. Currently, it is being used as an instructional tool to facilitate reading through the development of decoding skills, writing through the development of spelling and word study skills, and speech through the development of speech perception and articulation. Visual Phonics is neither a language nor a communication system; it is an instructional tool.

vocabulary: The words we must know to comprehend and communicate effectively. It includes oral vocabulary and reading vocabulary.

W

word consciousness: Refers to an awareness of and interest in words, their meanings, and their power and involves both a cognitive and an affective perspective toward words.

working memory: Also called *short-term memory*, it refers to a limited-capacity mental system responsible for the temporary storage and processing of information necessary to handle tasks that require comprehension, learning, and reasoning. It is a storage and processing system for modality-specific information.

writing vocabulary: The words we use in writing.

AUTHOR INDEX

SUBJECT INDEX

NOTE: Page numbers accompanied by *t* refer to table.